Baby Boomers Almanac™

How to attain, secure, and enjoy your three most important assets

"The great thing in this world is
not so much where we are, but
in what direction we are moving."

—*Oliver Wendell Holmes, Jr.*

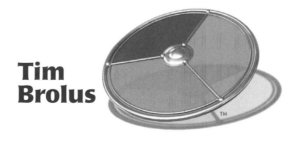

Tim Brolus

Better Living Publishing
MACOMB TOWNSHIP, MICHIGAN

First printing 2006
ISBN-13: 978-0-9778975-2-0
ISBN-10: 0-9778975-2-4
LCCN 2006923723

ATTENTION CORPORATIONS, UNIVERSITIES, COLLEGES, AND PROFESSIONAL ORGANIZATIONS: Quantity discounts are available on bulk purchases of this book for educational, gift purposes, or as premiums for increasing magazine subscriptions or renewals. Special books or book excerpts can also be created to fit specific needs. For information, please contact Better Living Publishing, Suite A, 45838 Rapids Drive, Macomb Twp, MI 48044; ph 586-228-1909; www.betterlivingpublishing.com.

Dedication

This book is dedicated to God, my family, and my peers, who have inspired, motivated, and empowered me never to give up on my dreams and life vision—and to share what I have lived and learned along the way to help others find more joy and relevance in their own lives.

Acknowledgment

This book could never have been written without the encouragement of my wife and peers. Their prodding of me to write about what is inside of me based on my experience was invaluable. Additionally, the help of one of my concept editors, Mary Kelley of Innovative Business Services, LLC, gave the ideas form. The wisdom and input of my wife and colleagues, along with Mary's extensive writing and organizational skills, showed me that the material had relevance. In a world of "I will get to it" professionals, Mary, and the top-notch team at About Books, Inc., are the "doers" that "got to it" and helped me make my vision a reality. And my wife...well she is a rare gem that adds dimension, value, and unconditional love to my life.

Disclaimer

The information in this book is designed for informational and educational purposes only. It is not intended to treat, diagnose, or prescribe any medical condition. It is not meant to replace the advice of your health care professional. Consult with your healthcare provider before using any of this information. It is merely a guide, an almanac, of what the "experts" tell us we can do not only to prolong our lives, but also to enjoy ourselves more in the process. It is sold with the exclusive understanding that the author and the publisher are not liable for the misconception or misuse of the information provided. Further, the author and Better Living Publishing shall have neither the liability, nor the responsibility to any person or entity with respect to any loss, damage, or injury caused or alleged to be caused directly or indirectly by the information or use of any product or service mentioned in this book.

Foreword

Consider this:

If you were to base your age on how old you feel...how old would you be?

If you were to measure your level of life satisfaction so far...where would you be on a scale of 1 to 10?

Further, if you don't like your answers to either, or both, of these questions...what would you be willing to do to get more of what you want and less of what you are unhappy with?

Like you, I am a part of the generation that "had all the answers" and vowed to stay young forever! I am a "baby boomer"—one of eighty-four million Americans born between 1946 and 1964. As I approach a major milestone—fifty years—I realize I *won't* stay young forever but I *do* have a few more decades to live (thanks to science), and I want to enjoy each of them to the max!

The premature death of my father, mother, and brother taught me that in order to plan for your future you must deal with your present and past. As a successful executive, business owner, former competitive bodybuilding champion, husband, and father, I am not going to just give in to premature aging. Are you? I want to stack the deck in my favor and maximize my body's chemistry to enjoy a robust, healthy, and rewarding life.

This book contains ten powerful sections for you to explore and apply to enhance your life. Read it from cover-to-cover, select a chapter at a time, or flip it open and put your new awareness into action each day.

Before you start, keep in mind that this is not about perfection or merely a collection of good ideas to add to your bookshelf. It's a way to simplify your life with a proven plan to get you from where you are to where you want to be in life. It will teach you how to make new choices that will have an immediate and profound effect on the quality of your health-span, wealth-span, and lifespan.

I'm not ready to throw in the towel just because I've had another birthday. Are you? We have life to live, roads to travel, and things to accomplish. Our work is not done...we are the Anti-Aging Baby Boomer Generation!

Are you ready to transform your life? Join me on a journey to take your life to a new level of relevance and value. Here's to planning the rest of your life.

After all, who wants to live longer if it's no fun?

> **"And in the end, it's not the years in your life that count. It's the life in your years!"**
> —Abraham Lincoln

Table of Contents

Introduction

The premature death of my father, mother, and brother from *lifestyle*-related disease, taught me that even though there are no guarantees in life, our future is purchased by the present—that your future life experience is impacted by how well you currently balance and integrate three key areas:

- ☻ **Your Body/Mind/Spirit Connection**
- ☻ **Your Relationships**
- ☻ **Your Finances**

I saw how a weakness or imbalance in any one—or all—of these areas leads to weakness, disease, misery, and death. And for the first time in my life, I experienced, first-hand, the importance of being brutally honest with myself about what I know and what I don't know… and how to fill in the gaps between the two.

How are you living the trilogy? On a scale of one to ten, how strong are you in these areas? How well are they integrated and balanced in your life? What's missing or needs to occur to make them a ten, both individually and collectively? What changes will you make and why? Your answers will either keep things as they are, let them erode further, or move you closer to a stronger and more rewarding life.

What's your vision for the future? Creating the life you want requires that you create a personal power plan that

1

integrates your vision for your future with your habits and removes the barriers to your success.

Your habits are like an interlinked web. Making a positive change in one area of your life automatically enhances another. When all three dimensions change at the same time, the results can be life-transforming—empowering you to enjoy more health and wellness care instead of sick care.

For example: a single change, such as physical exercise, can reduce body fat, increase lung capacity as well as muscle mass, lower cholesterol, reduce your heart rate, enhance self-esteem, redirect tension, and improve your immune system—all of which, in the end, can also save you money and preserve your wealth. One change impacts multiple body systems.

The fact is, the habits you have, or develop from this day forward, ultimately determine how your life unfolds.

> **"Life is like a combination lock; your job is to find the right numbers, in the right order, so you can have anything you want."**
> —Brian Tracy

That Was Then, This Is Now

Baby boomers have a history of challenging the norm, pioneering new thinking, and rarely accepting things at face value. So there is no need for any of us to accept the outmoded notions regarding our aging process.

Consider the impact we have had on society and culture over the years.

We didn't just eat food. We helped create the fast food industry's market, and, most recently, health and sports nutrition and medical spas.

2

We didn't just wear clothes. We transformed fashion and design with denims, bellbottoms, and polyester.

We didn't just get married. We broke the sexual and relationship taboos established in our parents' day.

We didn't just go to work. We transformed the workforce, breaking the pattern of lifetime employment and demanding women's equality in a male-dominated workforce.

And now we are once again making new decisions that defy convention regarding our health, value to society, and attitudes towards aging.

We Are Setting New Trends

We are in the midst of a longevity revolution—stopping the clock and rewriting the rules of retirement with a vision for something more exhilarating than a gold watch or time to play cards. We are becoming active participants in our future, as opposed to passive spectators—we're not going to be quitting and knitting.

We are at a social tipping point due to longer life spans, economic uncertainties, and mass rejection of yesterday's view of "getting old." This tipping point has compelled us to rethink our views concerning longevity. We are seeing the value that our wisdom, knowledge, and energy bring to our society. The new paradigm being embraced by the boomer generation includes:

- Lifelong education-pursuit of second, third, and even fourth careers
- Volunteerism
- Activism/championing causes dear to our hearts
- Seeking new and better methods for creating and sustaining wellness

We're transforming our futures as our generation has come to realize we have a number of decades—*not days*—left to live and be productive. Contrary to previous generations who used to stop working, go home, slow down, and die, what we want and are doing is once again setting us apart.

> **"Retirement at sixty-five is ridiculous. When I was sixty-five I still had pimples."**
>
> —George Burns

New Things on the Horizon:
How the Longevity Revolution Will Transform Our Lives

In the past, we use to die before our bodies wore out. We rarely concerned ourselves with lifestyle planning past our fiftieth birthday. But now, according to *Newsweek*, "Many don't expect to die....We expect to be cured" (11/14/05). In fact, according to a recent study by Merrill Lynch, the two biggest fears of baby boomers are:

- Being sick
- Not being able to pay for it...both ahead of "dying"
- Living longer, without breaking down, is a now a *bigger concern* than "dying"!

As a result, we are embracing new attitudes, lifestyles, and options. We are pushing the aging envelope by utilizing a new arsenal of tools that revive our "youthful" vitality and make life better. These tools include:

- Nutriceuticals, engineered with macro and micro nutrients to fight aging

♠ Cosmeceuticals for rejuvenation therapies that act like age erasers for both men and women

♠ Anti-aging spas

♠ Lifelong learning

♠ High-tech exercise gear programmed to train your body precisely to be stronger, healthier, and more youthful

♠ Manmade replacement body parts, from livers, kidneys, and lungs, to bone tune-ups

Some experts say that over seventy percent of our longevity is based on our habits and lifestyle. Use the following ten steps to reclaim your life, physically, mentally, emotionally, and/or financially, from the events, influences, and habits that accelerate your aging. Use them to create a new vision of who you want to be.

Let's start at the source…your thoughts.

Step #1:
Get Your Head in the Game

Get Back to *Your* ABCs...A + B = C
Attitude + Behavior = Current Life Experience

You only have control over two things in life—how you think and how you act. How you use these two things determines your life experience. They either build or destroy the life you want to enjoy.

There is no need to become a lesser version of yourself just because you've had another birthday.

> "The greatest revolution of our generation is the discovery that human beings, by changing the inner attitudes of their minds, can change the outer aspects of their lives."
> —William James

Perception Is Everything... Re-frame How You See Things

Whether you believe William James (we alter our lives by altering our thinking) or prefer Abraham Lincoln (we are as happy as we make our minds up to be) or relate to

Gandhi (you must become the change you want to see in the world)…the truth is the same. We change what we experience by changing what we believe, expect, and do. Everything you experience today is the result of the choices you've made in the past. If you don't like what you're getting from your life today, you need to change what you're doing—or not doing—to cause that which you don't like.

> "The definition of insanity is continuing to do the same thing, and expecting different results."
> —Anthony Robbins

How Old Is Old?
Is It Time for a New "AHA" (Attitude for Healthy Aging)

We tend to see things as we were told or taught to see them…not necessarily how they *could* be. As we increase our lifespan, the only way to increase our health and wealth span is to stop looking at our future potential with yesterday's eyeballs—the old rules just don't apply. We need to be open to expanding our capacity by changing the mindset and routines that brought us to this point…and rebuild some beliefs, goals, and actions based on the direction we want our life to be going from this point forward.

Are you getting better or bitter each birthday? Are you on top of your game or running on empty and ready to crash? Where you stand in life is the result of the accumulation of the thinking that brought you there. What were you *taught* to believe regarding your:

- Attitude and Beliefs
- Stress
- Nutrition
- Fitness
- Relationships
- Dreams, Goals, and Getting What You Want
- Spiritual Factor
- Financial Security

Did you ever consider that those "truths" are contributing to your current situation and future potential—good or bad? What about those mental maps and formulas, created over time, which define:

- How things are
- How things should be
- How to get there

The best way to test the value of thoughts, beliefs, or actions is to look at the results they are producing. Do they work *for* or *against* you? Are they bringing you closer to or further from what you want? Do they enhance your life or detract from it? Results don't lie. You either have what you want out of your life or you don't. If not, what changes are required to get what you want? My mentor shared several years ago a truth that is the foundation of all I do, so I will share it with you to apply to your own thought process:

You can't change the way things are with the same thinking that got you there in the first place.

What would happen if you had a new picture of how things could be and a new map of how to get there? One fueled by new ideas and truths to live on purpose instead of by chance, removing the barriers and brakes to your full potential?

Awareness and Empowerment Lead to New Realities

Your potential to live a vibrant and fulfilling life is tremendous. But nothing changes until you do. You, and you alone, hold the keys to your future. When you can link this "cause and effect" in your own life, you give birth to a new day. Instead of saying, "life" or "they" did this to me, you can say, "I did that to me, and therefore I can undo it!" You begin to realize the extraordinary power of personal choice in creating the life you want. By doing so, you can move beyond blame and choose to build an age-defying "personal empowerment" mindset—one that allows you to see and act on the fact that you either create or allow everything that happens to you. When things don't turn out as planned, you ask, "What can I do differently next time?"

> **"We are what we repeatedly do."**
> —Aristotle

With this mindset, you begin to take charge of your life, by realizing that you determine:
- What you eat and drink
- If, or how, you exercise
- How you rest or recreate your life
- What you believe
- How you think

For example, you:

- Told yourself "maybe it will go away" but never sought out help.
- Didn't say no to _____ and ignored the "yellow alerts" that said, "Caution, this is not right!"
- Chose what you read, what you listen to, who you "hang out" with, and what you watch on TV.
- Assumed "no news is good news" instead of looking into it.
- Accepted what you read, or heard, instead of checking out the facts.
- Did or didn't buy the _____, which would have helped you with_____.
- Bought the fitness book or membership but didn't start or stick with it.
- Decided "I don't need help and "went it alone!"
- Said you were too busy to _____.
- Thought you could never learn to budget or understand finances.
- Made excuses for why you skipped recommended wellness exams, or screenings…And on and on.

And these choices have created your life as it is today.

Endless New Possibilities

The only way to re-create your life, to enjoy the future you want, is to look at how you cause things to happen to you… either by what you do or fail to do. Until you focus on the cause and more importantly realize that *you* are the cause of what you're unhappy with, you're simply dancing on the surface of life—hoping and praying that "something is going to change." Remember, you can either be the victim of your life and let things happen to you, or you can be the master of your anti-aging mindset and you do things to create the life you desire.

Continually challenge what you hear or believe to determine if it adds up for you. This is not negative. It's simply a call for questioning a thought or belief for better ways of handling a particular situation.

This simple story may illuminate the point:

A man and his son are in a serious car accident. The father is killed, and the son is rushed to the closest emergency room. Upon arrival, the attending doctor looks down at the child and cries out, "This is my son!"

Question: Who is the doctor?

Unless you've heard this before, chances are you may be stumped. In order to solve this insight puzzle, you need to challenge the automatic assumption that all doctors are men—which, of course, they are not. The doctor is the boy's mom.

Continually questioning your perceptions is vital because it affects how you "see" everything in your world and how you "respond" to it. If your assumptions are inaccurate, then the behavior that follows will be the same…and that's not going to serve you well. Remember, in computer processing they say "garbage in, garbage out." The same concept applies to how well you age.

Heads or Tails—
Time for an Attitude Audit?

Like a two-sided coin, we are both optimists and pessimists. Some days we feel the world is out to get us, whereas others we can't wait to see what it has in store for us. Your mental habits determine your outcomes. In the words of the late Flip Wilson: "What you see is what you get…."

If you don't like your current life experience, pay attention to your responses to the events in your life. As optimists, we are conscious of both sides of the situation but choose to focus on the positive. This is not a naïve belief that life is only positive...it's just an awareness that we always have a choice as to how we think or act, so we can create more positive outcomes along the way.

Consider how the following scenario can stifle your ultimate life experience:

A husband is discussing with his wife how his clothes seem to be shrinking because they are fitting tighter. 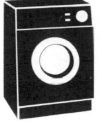 "Honey," says the husband, "please stop putting my pants in the dryer...they are shrinking!" She responds to her husband, "I think you have the wrong appliance; it's the refrigerator not the dryer we need to avoid."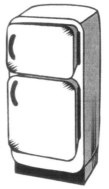

The problem here lies in the fact that the husband is looking "outside" himself for answers to his problems and concerns instead of *within* himself.

> "You can't do *everything* with a positive attitude, but you can do *anything* better!"
>
> —Zig Ziglar

Dare to Make a Fully Conscious Choice

Each and every thought and action has a ripple effect on how we feel and live. Ultimately, our life's path is determined by the sum of our personal choices. Consider this: If you don't like apples, but I give you $100 to eat an apple, would you find enough motivation to eat it? I wasn't born loving to exercise, eating right, and thinking in a more positive, un-stressful manner.

Losing my dad (from heart disease), my brother (from a stress disease), and my mom (from cancer) motivated me to take a critical look at my own beliefs, lifestyle, and goals. I saw a need for a change and adopted new habits and priorities to steer me in the direction of the life I desired.

What will be your reason, your motivator, your internal "why" factor to make some changes in *how* you live your life? What is the *one* thing that inspires you, at a root level, to start and stick with the habits and routines required to keep you from breaking down before you can leave a legacy? What will make taking better care of yourself a new, top priority—will it be money, family, career, your health…God?

If you want to change some things in your life, you need to change some things in your life.

The first change I made was to take a look at and act on my answers to these key questions:

- ☻ What do I want out of my life…why…and when?
- ☻ How am I creating or allowing the things currently taking place in my life—positive and negative?
- ☻ What's working that I need to do more of?
- ☻ What's not working that I need to stop doing or do less of—results don't lie!

Then, I developed a clear picture of what I wanted, and why…and wrote it down. I learned that seeing my ideas and options in writing helped me to picture my plans. It crystalized my thoughts and helped me to set new priorities. Finally, I created an action plan and committed to it—ushering in the support of a friend to keep me accountable.

How to Build a Better Life

Define *what* you want out of life in the next 1–5 years, 5–10 years, and 10–15 years. Identify *why* you want this …the difference it will make and the

If you are ready to enjoy a vibrant and rewarding life, realize that it doesn't happen by chance.

consequence(s) of doing nothing.

Then, commit to what you will do to get there. What do you need to start, stop, do more of, or less of? What is the first step you will take to get there, based on your personal *priorities*?

> "You cannot change circumstances, the seasons, or the wind, but you can change yourself"
>
> —Jim Rohn

Take a look at the chart that follows as an example of how others have built their "better life" list. To build yours, take a clean sheet of paper and create a chart of what you want, why, and what you'll do differently to get there, using specific ideas you get from the remaining sections of this book. Making one or two improvements a month will add up—bringing you over a dozen new weapons to build greater health, joy, and financial security into your coming years. Be careful not to take on too much too fast. It will only frustrate and discourage you from getting what you want.

I Want *More*...	Benefit: Because I Want *Fewer*...	So I Will...	Starting
Energy	Missed Opportunities		
Wellness	Eroding Health and Medical Bills		
Balance	Conflict and Feeling Overwhelmed		
Sense of Purpose	Meaningless Moments and Memories		
Better Memory	Mistakes		
Deeper Relationships	Detachment and Feeling Alone		
Restful Sleep	Tired Days		
Focus	Wasted Time and Chaos		
Confidence	Dissatisfaction		
Self-Esteem	Self-Acceptance and Embarrassment		
Joy	Regrets		
Happiness	Blah Days		
Time for My Dreams	Discontent		
Self-Approval	Self-Depreciation		
Stamina	Fatigue and Weakness		
Financial Security	Risk and Loss from Insecurity		

Now, take your new commitment to a better you and drop out of the "ain't it awful to get older club." Be the change you want to see in everyone else!

> **"It's time to start living the life you've imagined."**
>
> —Henry James

Step #2:
Deal with the Stressors in Your Life!

What do the following have in common:

- ♠ **You win the lottery**
- ♠ **You eat or skip a meal**
- ♠ **You go to or avoid the gym**
- ♠ **You relocate where you live**
- ♠ **Your best friend dies**

…Stress! They are all a type of stress.

Are you ready to challenge your thinking? Stress itself is not bad, and it is not always mental or emotional. Stress is part of life. It comes in many forms—physical, emotional, mental, and financial. The physical things you do to your body through diet and exercise can be just as tough on it as a mental or emotional strain. In other words, what you eat, drink, and breathe can be as harmful as what's eating you. For now we'll focus on the mental and emotional factors that cause unhealthy stress in your life.

Some mental and emotional stress is good for you. It pumps you up, gives you energy, and supplies zest for life. It "turns you on." Other stress, *dis*-stress, gnaws away at you and zaps your energy over the years. It wears you out. The thing to look for is how hard it hits, how long it lasts, and the time between its return.

Stress management is not, as it is commonly assumed, the process of getting rid of stress. Rather, the core role of stress management is becoming aware of your sources of stress and any accompanying symptoms and then choosing a solution to neutralize their negative impact on your body and mind with the following mindset:

- ☮ Here's what's happening
- ☮ Here's how it's affecting me
- ☮ Here's what I am committed to do about it

Practicing this three-part self-talk helps you to respond more positively to your environment and other stressors around you with less mental drain and wear or tear on your body.

By changing your perception, re-labeling your experiences, and building your body's resistance factors through proper diet, exercise, and holistic therapies, you can lessen the effects of personal distress. The result of those choices determines whether stress is your friend or foe.

> **"Your thinking alone, determines if life sharpens your edge or grinds you down to dust."**
> —Anonymous

Stress manifests itself differently depending on the individual. Some feel wired or tired, whereas others feel depressed or burnt out and experience aches and pains.

Some common warning signs that stress is taking its toll are: a persistent negative mood, difficulty relaxing, occasional sleeplessness, neck or back pain, and overall lack of a sense of well-being.

According to the American Academy of Family Physicians and other stress specialists, some classic signs it is a foe are:

- ♠ Allergies
- ♠ Anger or hostility toward yourself or others
- ♠ Angina
- ♠ Anxiety
- ♠ Apathy or lack of initiative
- ♠ Back pain
- ♠ Chronic coughs or frequently reoccurring respiratory ailments
- ♠ Constipation or diarrhea
- ♠ Craving salt or foods high in salt
- ♠ Decreased sexual drive or performance
- ♠ Depression
- ♠ Environmental sensitivities or allergies
- ♠ Fatigue
- ♠ Frequently occurring infections
- ♠ Frequent sighing or gasping for breath
- ♠ General irritability most of the time
- ♠ Grinding of teeth
- ♠ Headaches or tension that won't go away
- ♠ High blood pressure
- ♠ Inability to concentrate or remember things: e.g., "Where are my keys?"
- ♠ Inability to relax
- ♠ Inability to feel rested, no matter how much sleep you get
- ♠ Insomnia
- ♠ Low blood sugar
- ♠ Multiple signs and symptoms with no medical diagnosis

- Muscle aches
- Panic attacks
- Problems with relationships
- Shortness of breath
- Thoughts of self-destruction
- Upset stomach
- Weight gain or loss

Can too little stress be bad? Absolutely. Lack of change or stimulation in your job or daily routine can adversely affect your quality of life. The key is to keep balance in your lifestyle and habits to ease the negative effects of stress and prevent the vast array of related health issues from *dis*-ease.

What makes mental and emotional stress friend or foe?

***Frequency*:** How often does it occur?

***Intensity*:** How do you react and how does your body compensate?

Time: When does it occur and how long does it last?

***Type*:** What's the source...your thoughts, environment or lifestyle, relationships?

So what can you do?

Use these StressBusters® to stop stressing and start living better.

Stressorcise #1:
Harvest Some Happiness

In Section One, you were asked to get your "head in the game." The next question is, "How are you using your head to fight stress?" What you think about affects your body. Think about a lemon, and your mouth fills with saliva. Ponder your worries, and your body produces stomach acid. Focus on your anger and fear, and your body sounds the hormone alarm, to "fight or flee!"

Every situation is a chance to change the mind. Those attached to their mental position resist this concept because they fear the consequences of uncertainty. In truth, fear comes from anticipating the future and feeling unprepared. Master your thoughts, and you start to master negative stress.

> **"You are today where your thoughts have brought you; you will be tomorrow where your thoughts take you."**
> —James Allen, author of
> *As A Man Thinketh*

- ☙ Start by creating a positive expectation.
- ☙ Plant positive thoughts.
- ☙ Nurture yourself and your relationships with positive self-talk.
- ☙ Protect yourself from mental pollution of others—passing on guilt, abuse, or denial, etc.
- ☙ Watch your "personal computing"…look at how you perceive things and process them.
- ☙ Don't "soil" yourself with dirt in the form of "shoulds" …don't let anyone "should on you" anymore.
- ☙ Allow yourself to let go of the need to control every outcome, every time. People with control issues are fearful of unknown outcomes.

21

> **"Laughter is like changing a baby's diaper—it doesn't solve any problems permanently, but it makes things more acceptable for a while."**
> —Anonymous

One way to build a more positive life for yourself is to modify how you react to your emotions or the emotions of others. Every emotion has value—even sadness and disappointment. Realize, however, that our emotions are not our life. They are our reaction to it.

Patience…something you admire in the car behind you, but not in the one in front of you.

Learn how to let your emotions build your life *rather* than destroy it. Keep in mind what we learned at the crossing guard's corner on the way to school: *stop, look, and listen!*

- ♣ ***Stop***, and scan your body for stored tension (clenched teeth, tight hands, rapid breathing, etc.).
- ♣ ***Look*** at the situation rationally—do you need to reframe what you are seeing in a different light?
- ♣ ***Listen*** to your inner voice and modify how you react to your emotions or the emotions of others.
- ♣ ***Proceed*** with caution…and don't stay in the middle of the road; you may get run over!

Here's a power tip: Know that *whatever you judge…you attract or become.*

For Example: If you're arrogant, continually putting down, judging, or criticizing others, you'll find you will draw the same experiences into your own life. Your words and actions will create an equal or greater reaction out of others. Hence, the popularity of the phrases: "Takes one to know one" and "Birds of a feather flock together."

> **"You are a living magnet. What you attract in your life, is in harmony with your dominant thoughts."**
> —Brian Tracy

Magnetize your mental magnets—ask the right questions, and watch your world get better.

Improving your outer world begins by redesigning your relationship with yourself. What you say in the privacy of your own mind determines what life says back to you. My mom used to say, "Don't be like the pot calling the kettle black." Before you try to change your relationship with others, listen to your inner voice. What is it saying to you throughout your day?

- Why me?
- Seek and destroy?
- Conquer or connect?
- My way or the highway!
- In order to make me right, I need to make you wrong!
- Is it defining this moment as an "urgency" or emergency?
- Is it measuring your life in thankfulness or worthiness?
- Do you practice self-forgiveness or have an attitude that "nothing less than perfect is acceptable!"
- Is the glass half full or half empty?
- Does it propel you to live some cause greater than self?
- Are you addressing your shortcomings and magnifying your strengths…or promoting destructive self-talk and criticism?

Telling yourself any one of these thoughts is a tip-off to stop your mind for a moment, look inside, and ask *"How can I create better thoughts? How can I surround myself with the right people?"* Consider seeking out a mentor as a shoulder to lean on to challenge you to make better decisions through better thoughts. A psychologist once shared with me that the best measurement tool for the value of any thought and action is:

> **Something is good to the degree to which it fulfills its purpose.**

The question we must ask is, "Does the end justify the means?" For example, let's say you want to lose fifteen pounds and go on a diet. If the purpose of dieting is simply to lose weight and you lose weight, it worked. However, if your goal is to improve your energy and health, *while* you shed those pounds—and your program makes you skinny and sick—then you must match your actions to your ultimate goal…which is both to look and feel your best.

Whether it's weight control and health or anything else, make sure to match your plan to your goal—not just some short-term result.

Other "happiness harvesters"—eliminate self-limiting beliefs from your mindset such as:

- ♣ *Insecurity:* "I can't stoop to that job."
- ♣ *Denial:* "As long as I stay busy, I must be making good progress."
- ♣ *Excess pride:* "I know what I am doing, because I do it all the time."
- ♣ *Fear:* "I can't do it…what if they don't like me or it doesn't work?"

Try this exercise to erase self-limiting beliefs. For the next seven days, write down any thought you have that limits your value on a piece of paper and collect the slips in an envelope or basket. Once a week, light a candle and cautiously but deliberately burn each individual slip in a meaningful, symbolic ceremony—announcing aloud that these thoughts are no longer a part of who you are.

Put your past behind you. Do the same exercise above with a different purpose. Write down your regrets—the lost loved ones, broken relationships, neglected hobbies, ruined investments, bungled education, all the opportunities that blew away—and flush them down the toilet. As you see them leave your hand and go down the drain, go on with your day feeling the renewed energy from having them flushed from your life.

> "There is no right or wrong, only our thinking makes it so."
> —Abraham Lincoln

Stressorcise #2:
Tame Your Tension

If you find most stress-reduction techniques too time consuming or impractical when you need relief the most, try this simple do-anywhere technique. The same internal voice that told you to get upset in an instant can tell you to relax. Perhaps it's a discouraging moment on the phone, lengthy lines in the bank, or rush-hour traffic that allows stress to get to you—know your triggers so you can be proactive and detour around destructive stress whenever possible.

Practice the following exercise a few times and feel free to add some variation of your own. Close your eyes and repeat to yourself: "I…am…relaxed… I…am… relaxed." Now picture a car's speedometer at 80 mph. Watch it fall: 70, 60, 50, 40, 30, 20, and stop it there. Repeat: "I…am…relaxed" as you open your eyes slowly. Don't practice while driving however!

Another variation: Visualize an elevator button system. Start at the twentieth floor and go down to the second floor in the same way you reduced the speed on your speedometer.

Intervene: *steal* more time from tension using these simple techniques.

Silence your stressors by putting problems on pause with the "Quieting Response."

Stop what you are doing for a moment. Close your eyes, if possible. Drop your shoulders as you take a slow and deep breath in through your nose for a count of ten.

Exhale, while saying to yourself, or, out loud if you are alone, "I am calm and relaxed" …and feel the tension melting your arms, legs, face, neck, and back each time you exhale.

Repeat three times, go on with your day, and feel the tension drain from your brain, shoulders, neck, and body as you fill up with vitalizing energy from oxygen. (Remember to breathe for the rest of the day.)

Deep Breathing for Deep Relief

How often do you pay attention to your breathing? Like most habits, it's usually done unconsciously. Proper breathing is an integral part of defusing destructive stress. Poorly oxygenated blood contributes to depression, fatigue, anxiety, and other stressful states. During the day you might catch yourself yawning or sighing. During stressful times you may find yourself losing your wind. A sigh, yawn, or loss of breath is the body's signal that it needs more oxygen (hypoxia) or feels tension.

All too often we breathe shallowly or hyperventilate during stress because of habit... Reconditioning yourself to take full, deep breaths during both stressful and relaxed times is valuable. Here's how:

- ◑ Sit or stand up straight.
- ◑ Sigh deeply, letting out a sound of deep relief as air rushes out of your lungs.
- ◑ Don't think about inhaling—just let the air come in naturally.
- ◑ Exhale slowly.
- ◑ Now, think about deliberately filling your diaphragm and lungs with air. Push your stomach out.
- ◑ Exhale all three areas, starting with your chest, then diaphragm, and finally your stomach.

The Progressive Relaxation Technique

- ◑ Lie down and get yourself as comfortable as you can. Loosen or remove your shoes, ties, or belt.
- ◑ Become aware of your breathing (like we discussed above)...taking in slow, deep breaths through your nose, and exhale out through your mouth.

❧ Starting with your toes, tense your muscles for a count of ten and relax them for a count of ten, progressively working your way up your body (calves, knees, thighs, buttocks, stomach, back, shoulders, arms...chest...chin...mouth...face...and forehead). Feel the tension drain as you slowly release each area's tension.

Other Tension Releasers

During walks to your car after work or shopping, take your time. Then listen to your thoughts for signs of distress and extinguish them with the Quieting Response above.

Pause and stop between activities. Take two to three slow, deep breaths. When you get to the car, fill your body with energy and dissolve any building tension before you get behind the wheel.

Between roles (coming home from the work or gym, etc.) take time to change clothes to ease the transition into your next role.

You watch the clock, right? Then use it to unwind. Stick little colored dots on all your time pieces. Then, whenever you check them, you'll be reminded to practice a Quieting Response.

Rise and Shine

Instead of leaping for the shower...immediately after the alarm clock sounds, lie in bed quietly for a few moments, listening to your slow and rhythmic breathing, saying to yourself, I am calm and ready for my day. If you are spiritual, invoke a prayer of thankfulness and blessing upon the day and anyone you encounter in it.

Take a sanity break. While driving the car...turn off the radio and tune *into* body tension. Sit back and unclench your death grip on the wheel. Release the tension from your legs and shoulders.

Get a pet and walk it (great exercise), talk to it (a non-critical listener), hug it (it feels good), and care for it (it's nice to feel appreciated).

Stressorcise #3:
Remove Success Killers
and Attitude Traps

Sometimes our reaction to problems is worse than the problem. A good rule of thumb for reducing your tension from stress is to reduce the "threat messages" you send yourself. If a situation really poses a threat to something important to you, you'd be foolish to ignore it. You need to gear up when truly threatened. But when no threat exists, or when the issue simply isn't important, you're foolish to gear yourself up for an internal or external fight. Often, the way we perceive a problem *is* the problem.

Don't Worry Yourself to Death

Consider the story of Nick Sitzman, a strong and healthy man who worked the rail yards. He seemed to have everything: a strong ambition, a wife and two children whom he loved dearly, and many friends.

Nick, however, had one fault. He worried about everything and usually feared for the worst.

One summer day, the crew quit work early to celebrate the boss's birthday. While checking the rail cars, Nick was accidentally locked in one of the refrigerator cars, and the rest of the work crew left the work site.

Nick panicked. He banged and shouted for help until his fists were bloody and his voice was hoarse. No one heard him. His mind began to review his situation and options. He calculated that the temperature was about zero degrees. He thought, "If I can't get out, I'll freeze to death in here."

Wanting to let his wife and family know exactly what happened to him, Nick found a knife and began to etch words on the railcar floor. He wrote, "It's so cold, my body is getting numb. If I could just sleep. These could be my last words."

The next morning the crew slid open the heavy doors of the boxcar and found Nick dead. An autopsy revealed that every physical sign of his body indicated he had frozen to death. And yet, the refrigeration unit of the car was inoperative, and the temperature inside indicated fifty-five degrees. Nick had killed himself by the power of worry.

What he presumed to be a dangerous event was later revealed to pose no real threat to his well-being.

The Cost of Your Reaction

Although you may not find yourself in a locked rail car, be careful not to kill yourself with your thoughts. Your basic beliefs dictate your response to potentially stressful events in your life. Learn to deal with your problems by asking yourself, does a real problem exist, or is the problem one of *perception*?

For example, have you ever fought for a place in line or to make your point during a meeting or discussion when you knew your actions or feelings wouldn't make a difference, but you just wanted to be heard? If so, you know what it is like to spend ten dollars worth of adrenalin on a ten cent problem.

I recently saw two people actually live this example while I waited to get on the freeway. I was the third person in line at the light to enter the freeway. I noticed the first person was not moving even though it was a green light. The second person was honking and yelling. The first person got out of his car and said:

> "I'll hold your horn if you'll start my car."

31

Be on guard that your style of thinking doesn't deplete your energy and reserves, leaving you out of gas and unable to take action when you really need to.

How about "Under-Reacting"?

When confronted by a threat or situation you consider important (such as discipline with children or acting to stop a disintegrating relationship), you'd be foolish just to remain detached, watch objectively, and do nothing…keeping your head in the sand. In this case you need to respond to avoid unnecessary loss.

To use your stress energy appropriately, aim to spend the amount of energy appropriate for the importance of the situation and the degree of threat. Get better at spending ten cents worth of energy on ten-cent problems and one hundred dollars on a hundred-dollar problem. Think about how you could budget your stress energy differently. Stop for a moment and think of a couple of recent reactions in two areas:

- ☣ Today, this week, this month…how many times and in what situations have I spent ten dollars worth of adrenalin on a one-hundred-dollar problem or vice versa?
- ☣ Remind yourself to adjust your reactions with new awareness.

The goal is to stop playing the "would've, should've, could've" game and move on with greater awareness toward your ultimate goals.

Keep in mind, however, dealing with your life struggles may require that you to look deeper for their cause. You can start this process by answering some of the ultimate questions of life, such as:

- ♣ **Where is my life going? (your goals)**
- ♣ **What is important to me? (your values)**
- ♣ **What are my beliefs? (your faith) and who am I? (your self concept)**

Let your beliefs, values, and goals be the basis for saying "yes" to some things, and "just say no" to others.

Other Attitude Traps

You can be your own stumbling block or a springboard to the things you want in life. Psychologists say that three things help to determine on which side of the fence you fall.

- ♣ Your attitude toward change
- ♣ "ANTs"—Automatic Negative Thoughts
- ♣ Self-limiting beliefs

Change is a part of life. When it occurs, you can either accept it or reject it. Accepting it means you view it as a way to make your life richer, easier, and more rewarding. Resisting it, however, results in being run over by its sheer momentum. To help embrace any change, ask two questions:

- ♣ What's the payoff if I keep things as they are?
- ♣ What's the cost I will keep paying for keeping things as they are?

ANT control! Do you usually focus on the negatives in your life? In his book, *Change Your Brain, Change Your Life,* Daniel Amen, MD, shares that one of the things limiting our quality of life is the "ANTs" (Automatic Negative Thoughts) in our lives. One of the most deadly ANTs for baby boomers is "blaming."

When we blame, we live our life as a victim instead of enjoying it as an incredible journey. To enjoy more and fret less in life, stop blaming others for your lot in life. Assume full responsibility for the events that go on around you. Doing so keeps you from being a puppet on a string to anyone or anything.

Other "ANTs" to look for and rid yourself of are:

- Thinking in terms of "always" or "never." Using other words that dictate extreme absolutes such as: "everyone," "no one," "every time," and "everything," etc.

- Focusing on the negative: Your mind is your biggest critic of yourself and others. You focus on and talk about how bad your life is. The world is against *you!*

- Fortune-telling: I call this one "borrowing trouble." Your inner voice is constantly interpreting and telling you what people are thinking, why they do what they do, worrying they are mad at you or against you—and you end up entirely misreading them.

- Guilt beating: Thinking with words such as "should," "must," "ought to," or "have to," etc..

- Thinking with your feelings—Woe is *me!* No one cares if I live or die!

- Labeling: A self-righteous mindset that lumps yourself or others into a category without making any allowances for your differences. You use expressions like they are such ____(bums, idiots, cold-hearted people, etc.).

- Personalizing—When you put a personal meaning on a neutral event, such as why someone hasn't called you in a while, saying things like, "They must be mad at me."

As you can see, like pesky little picnic pests, ANTs can be very destructive in your life. But they don't have to be. *Here is a three-step plan to keep them from ruining your life experience:*

- Become aware of them.

- Shake them off or stomp them out!
- Stop the invasion. Remove them from your thoughts, replacing them with more affirming thoughts.

For more help on the matter, pick up a copy of Dr. Amen's book and stomp out these annoying pests.

Stop the domino effect. We all have bad days. It's part of life. The point is, don't let your bad day become a bad week, month, year, or life! When you catch yourself giving excuses like, "Well, I came from a bad home…" as the reason for your current life misfortune, it's time for an attitude adjustment.

You *are* capable of enjoying no limits living. Life coaches tell us that a feeling of "unworthiness" is one of the most pervasive limiting beliefs in baby boomers. Somehow we believe that we are incapable or not deserving of the best life has to offer. Look at the chart below to see if any of these limiting beliefs affects you. What is their impact on your life? How can you change things from the inside out?

What You Hear	How You Act on It Today in Life
Children should be seen and not heard	*I need to be quiet if I want love and approval*
Money doesn't grow on trees	*I'll never be wealthy and secure*
Get tough	*I'm weak*
You're so selfish	*My needs can wait*
Eat everything on your plate	*I can't waste this*
Nobody has ever made it as a _____	*Who am I kidding— why even try?*
You're so dumb	*Look what an idiot I am*
Act like a lady	*It's not okay to joke around or be sexy*
Your opinion doesn't matter	*What I think and say is worthless*

Here is a simple way to turn a limiting belief into an empowering one...

My limiting belief is _____

The way it limits me is _____

The way I want to be, act, or feel is _____ , *and it feels better this way.*

Step three is critical because it helps you purposely plant positive thoughts into your mind. Repeat this "new you" statement (affirmation) several times a day, for a month, and watch it "take root."

Survive or Thrive...Which Do You Want?

Vibrant boomers find that if they have enough faith, desire, determination, and persistence they can accomplish almost anything. But just because you're kicking up a lot of dust doesn't mean you're getting any closer to your goals. In his book, *The Art Of Living Consciously*, Nathanial Brandon shares the importance of keeping the following principles a priority in all of your pursuits for personal excellence:

- ♠ Determination
- ♠ Diligence
- ♠ Perseverance
- ♠ Consistency
- ♠ Integrity
- ♠ Professionalism
- ♠ Talent

Stressorcise #4:
Touch the Lives of Others
(and Better Your World)
While Building Relationships

Make your world a better place and give yourself a healthy jolt of self-esteem. Reaching out has a tremendous impact on how you feel about you…and ultimately how you relate to your world overall.

- Be a friend.
- Rekindle a long-lost childhood friendship.
- Become a mentor.
- Champion a cause.
- Share a hobby.
- Become a Big Sister/Big Brother.
- Make good art.
- Take risks.
- Nurture friendships.
- Blaze a new trail.

> **"Step Outside Yourself to See What's Important to Someone Else"**
> —Dale Carnegie

You may not have the power to solve the world's energy crisis, but each individual has the ability to take small steps that can have a big impact on their "world" and the community-at-large. You don't need a cape or a magic power to be a hero! One boomer I know decided to make cookies and write letters to our troops overseas. Even though the soldiers were strangers at first, they have now become an extended family bonded by a mutual respect and admiration for each other.

> "The things you remember most aren't always things."
> —Unknown

Take the Opportunity to Build Solid Friendships and Nurture Them Regularly

Researchers at the University of North Carolina at Chapel Hill found that holding hands and getting a hug releases a hormone, oxytocin, which helps lower blood pressure in women. *So take two hugs and call me in the morning.* In his book *121 Ways to Live 121 Years…And More,* Dr. Ronald Klatz, President of the American Academy of Anti-Aging Medicine, states that therapeutic touch helps relieve pain, depression, and anxiety.

> "Keep your family close and your friends even closer."
> —Dr. Ronald Klatz

Maximize Father Time

When my dad died suddenly from a heart attack, less than a year from my sixteenth birthday, he took with him all of the wisdom and knowledge we were both waiting for him to share. On the flip side, before my mom died several years later, she invested hundreds of hours of one-on-one time that helped to build the inner wealth I have today.

Children are our most valuable asset—and hold the key to our future. Invest time to build their inner wealth, whether they're your own or those that you mentor. Empower them with your knowledge, values, and beliefs. Regardless of the hand life has dealt you in the past, don't pass on your pain or hold back your time or energy. Equip them for life instead of handicapping them through neglect, apathy, or absence.

Corporate sales trainer Brian Tracy tells us that relationships that are not continually reinforced die. If business owners can make the effort to build relationships, in order to build their bank accounts, doesn't it make sense that we can do so to build the inner wealth of others as well as ourselves? I believe that the following quote from a poster I saw several years ago in a client's office really drives the point home: "A hundred years from now it will not matter what my bank account was, the sort of house I lived in, or the kind of car I drove...but the world may be different because I was important in the life of a child."

Plant a mother lode of inner wealth in the world around you. Make time today to reflect on what you want to contribute to the lives of your children and others...

- ☣ Take stock of your strengths and weaknesses
- ☣ Think about what hasn't worked in the last year
- ☣ Plan: "here is what I will do differently this year..."

Build up others every chance you get. And remember to tell those that you care about that you love them...because you never know if it will be your last time to share with them.

Consult these resources for help in deepening your personal relationships:

The Lessons of Love: Rediscover Our Passion for Life When It All Seems Too Hard to Take by Melody Beattie

Do You Know Your Husband? by Pam Carlinski

Do You Know Your Wife? by Pam Carlinski

How to Get Married After 35 by Helen Rosenberg, M.D.

Sex & Love for Grown Ups by Sallie Folley (rec by AARP)

How to Go On Living When Someone You Love Dies by Theresa Rando, Ph.D.

Getting the Love You Want: A Guide for Couples by Harville Hendrix, Ph.D.

Mars & Venus On a Date by John Gray

If you (or someone you love) is contemplating or facing divorce (a high-stress situation), consider *Spiritual Divorce* by Debbie Ford.

Stressorcise #5:
Manage Expectations

How many roles are you trying to fill each day: parent, brother, sister, leader, mentor, coach, boss, friend, teacher, etc. Does it seem like everyone wants a piece of you—even your pets? How do you cope with all these expectations? How do you avoid personal burnout when in the midst of a struggle between being everything for everyone else and still having something left for yourself?

Use this exercise to help avoid a crash:

♣ Start by writing out your various roles: parent, employer, employee, sibling, caregiver, etc.

♣ Clarify your top life priorities, goals, and expectations of each role.

♣ Create a "stop doing" list for yourself to set up some boundaries that stop you from going down a side road that could lead to a crash. For example, through the years of good/bad experiences, my list includes:

• I never lend my car. Too much room for unnecessary loss and conflict.

• I never lend money. If I give it, I do it freely…I'm not a bank.

• I never lend books. I'm not a library.

• I don't say "yes" when I mean "no." I want my intentions to be clear and honest.

• I don't over-commit myself outside my home. My family is my top priority.

To minimize the tension and strain from *multi*-role pile-ups, follow the air traffic controller's rule: "Land one plane at a time," as you:

♣ Verify if what you face is an emergency (can't wait) or an urgency (can wait).

♨ Pause to ask yourself: "What are my top life priorities? Is there another way to look at what I face? What single action can I take to get the outcome I desire?"

Don't limit your thoughts to "something has to go." Look for what to include, not exclude, to gain greater balance and self-control.

Maintain your composure by using the Quieting Response (Stressorcise #2) to redirect tension, relax your body, and clear your mind...*and take it with a sense of calm and confidence.*

Stressorcise #6:
Manage Your Self...Not Just Time

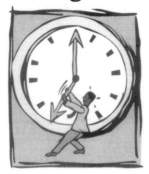

It is impossible to act in one area of life without it affecting your whole life. The way you use your time can increase or reduce your stress...*a lot*. Good self-managers reduce their stress levels by using many of the techniques listed below to manage their use of time...and ultimately themselves.

For starters—put a check next to those that you could use today:

- Create a "Top Five Tasks For Today" list each day.
- Make lists, isolate your top three priorities, and check items off when completed.
- Schedule your time more effectively. Allow time for travel and the unexpected.
- Use your peak energy time to do your hardest tasks.
- When you are interrupted, make a *decision* about what to do. Don't automatically "take" the interruption.
- Review how you spend your time—and note when you are most alert and creative (time for Essential Tasks) and assess how you can use your time more effectively tomorrow.
- Sort papers, then handle each piece only once.

To get the most impact from this list of self-management skills, ask yourself one penetrating question each time you are about to act:

"What one thing can I do...and only I do...that, if done now, and done right, will have the greatest impact on what I want at this time from myself and life?"

43

Reserve a daily "time out" to:

♠ Be still, relax, and clear your thinking.

♠ Sort tasks into three easy categories: Essential, Important, and Unimportant

♠ Ensure that your tasks include things that create balance and that they include things you like to do for yourself and things that will bring you closer to your life goals.

Get it done.

♠ Revisit the areas of your life that have a list of "incompletes."

♠ Ask yourself "what needs to be done to complete each task," and set up an action plan with a specific date to complete it and any resources you need to utilize or acquire to complete the task.

♠ Adjust your schedule (because your incompletes list is now a new priority) to get it done.

You'll find that *five things completed* brings you more value than a dozen things left undone.

> **"You will miss 100% of all the shots you don't take."**
> —Anonymous

Stressorcise #7: Recharge Your Battery— Jumpstart a New Attitude

Is there an area of your life that is not working out as well as you would like it to? Often, our attitude is the culprit, drawing more negative than positive energy into our life. But how do we learn to focus more on the negative than the positive in our lives—and not acknowledge the good in ourselves or others? According to Jack Canfield, co-creator of *Chicken Soup for the Soul*®:

> "In school, most of your teachers marked the answers you got wrong with an X rather than marking the ones you got right with a check mark or star. In sports, you got yelled at when you dropped the football or the baseball. There was almost more emotional intensity around your errors, mistakes, and failures than was around your successes."

One of my clients recently told me that her father used to grade her coloring, to teach her to stay inside the lines. Wow! Psychologists tell us that the more you acknowledge past success, in yourself and others, the more positive you are in your self-talk and conversations. They also recommend that instead of stewing over your flaws and the things you don't like, look at what you *do* like.

Attitudes are like muscles: The ones you use the most become the strongest. Strengthen your confidence, joy, and life value with the following "character push-ups":

- ♣ Smile…it's contagious.
- ♣ Practice a new way each day to be more cheerful and outgoing.
- ♣ Make a "Top Ten Best" list of your mate.
- ♣ List all the reasons you enjoy your job.

- List your top five strengths and find a way to practice them in the next twenty-one days.
- Practice forgiveness—go forty-eight hours without criticizing yourself or others.
- Catch others in the act—offering sincere praise to someone for a job well done.
- Pat yourself on the back for a job well done.
- Do a good deed without telling anyone.
- Follow through on one thing you have left unfinished.
- Be forgiving and eliminate grudges.
- Assume responsibility for something you've done wrong and make amends.
- Be honest with yourself and others about expectations.
- Begin with the end result in mind (a vision) instead of only the obstacles.
- "Count the cost" before you commit to a project or task.
- Seek to understand first, then to be understood.
- Practice patience today (with yourself and others!).
- Spend fifteen minutes today reading something to build greater balance.
- Write a personal letter or mission statement with what you like about yourself and why.
- Get a daily dose of sunlight and fresh air. Open the blinds and windows or, better yet, go for a walk.

Debrief Your Day—and Move Yourself Forward

It's easy to focus on the bad parts of our day. A great tool to focus on and reinforce the positive in your life is to create a daily Success Log. It's a great way to boost your confidence by making time daily to focus on the positive parts of your day that are moving you forward. Use the blank chart below to get started.

In the "what I did" section, list three things you accomplished today in various areas of your life, such as: healthy habits, career, family, work, community, spiritual, personal growth, finances, etc.

- ☸ Write in the next column why this was important and the benefit to you.
- ☸ In the third column, write in how you can keep positive momentum in this area of your life.
- ☸ Finally, fill in the next action you can take to enhance your progress in this area of your life.

Now, reinforce its positive value by reading it out loud before bed. If you have a family, be sure to tell them what you are doing so they don't think you're talking to the air around you.

Recently, a friend shared with me, "Sometimes I feel it's not a good day because *one* thing went wrong. There may have been good things as well, but the tendency is to focus on the *one* thing that went wrong. This process helps stop me from falling into a self-defeating rut and move on with greater."

Today's Successes

Day: _____ Date: _____

What I did	Why it was important	How to enhance	Next Step

Remember, your life journey is the result of your focus— you become what you "thought you would."

"I believe there are no mistakes in life as long as you learn the lessons. We all face challenges in our lives. For some it is cancer; for some it is alcohol; for some of us it is relationships. Those challenges are obstacles in our lives, put there for us to learn. The lesson may not be readily apparent. You will know you have learned the lesson when you can look back on the challenge as a gift."
—Dr. Michael Green

Stressorcise #8:
Call Upon Professionals to Help Eliminate Stored Tension

If you feel tightness in your shoulders, stiffness in your neck, or knots in your stomach, you're probably storing tension. *Make time to drain this tension and recuperate in a way that is meaningful to you.*

Massage therapies are widely recognized as effective forms of stress reduction. Studies in the Touch Research Institute of Florida show that the benefits of massage have quick results. Immediately after massage therapy sessions, subjects experienced a change in brain waves in the direction of heightened alertness and better performance on math problems (completed in less time with fewer errors).

In addition, massage therapy helps relieve muscular tension, revitalize energy, and strengthen your immune system—all of which contributes to reduced job stress and elevated moods. Other benefits include helping your body rid itself of stored toxins that adversely affect health and vitality. Body work may involve rubbing, kneading, and stroking of your body to ease stiffness, aches, and pains. In addition, the therapist may play soft, soothing music to enhance your ability to relax and have an emotional release from internal pain as well. Depending on your stress level, you may find it beneficial to make weekly, biweekly, or monthly appointments to receive treatments.

The ancient Taoists were renowned for their study of the arts of health and longevity. The gentle movements of Taoist Tai Chi convey the essence of this tradition to the modern world. Taoist Tai Chi is a gentle form of exercise that can be performed by anyone and benefit even those with advanced chronic conditions or those confined to a wheel chair. Regular practice of Taoist Tai Chi can bring a wide range of health benefits to the muscular, skeletal, and circulatory systems. The flowing movements of Taoist Tai Chi serve as a moving meditation that reduces stress and provides a way to cultivate body and mind. Tai Chi is offered at many community centers and through private lessons. Tai Chi videos and DVDs are also popular.

Many people think that yoga is stretching. But while stretching is certainly involved, yoga is really about creating balance in the body through developing both strength and flexibility. This is done through the performance of poses, each of which has specific physical benefits. Yoga teachers will often refer to "your practice," which means your individual experience with yoga as it develops over time. The amazing thing about yoga is that your practice is always evolving and changing, so it never gets boring. Yoga can be performed alone using a DVD or video or in a group.

Chiropractic Corrective Care also offers stress relief and other health benefits. Your spine and central nervous system are the control center for all functions of your body, so it makes sense to see a professional who specializes in the care and optimizing of these systems through a structured program of care. If you do choose a chiropractor, be sure he or she gives you *total solutions* to your unresolved health changes, not just a block of paid adjustments.

Dr. Gary Shoemaker, founder of Clairpointe Family Chiropractic, says you should expect a good chiropractor to offer you answers to:

Terminology…How do they explain:
- ♣ Chiropractic?
- ♣ Subluxation?
- ♣ Innate?

Adjustments...
- Why are they necessary?
- How is the frequency determined?
- Can you do it yourself?
- How do they explain your VSC (Vertibral Subluxation Complex) to you?

X-Rays...
- What are they used for?
- Are they safe?
- Why aren't they in color?

Cervical Extension Tractioning...
- How is it different from regular tractioning?
- When do I start, and how long does it last?
- What does it do?

Wellness...
- What is wellness?
- How do you get it?
- How do you keep it?

Diet, Exercise, and Supplements...
- When can I start exercising?
- Which supplements should I take?
- What's the best diet to use?
- How will they measure your success?

Other ways to redirect, release, and disengage from stored tension include:
- Counseling
- Spiritual Guidance
- Meditation
- Fitness Training or Pilates

Stressorcise #9: Stopping the Drain from Life's Surprises

I will never forget the moment I first heard that my mother was diagnosed *with cancer*. In the midst of her "exploratory surgery," the doctor came out and informed me and my sister, "She probably won't make it through the night." Ouch! Everything seemed so surreal. What will happen next? How will we make it? How will I handle the grief of her absence? My whole life seemed just to stop with this unwelcome surprise intrusion into my world.

No one likes surprises involving loss. In his book, *How to Stop Worrying and Start Living*, Dale Carnegie shares a simple but effective exercise to tame your worry and energize your life. Next time you find yourself in the midst of a "sucker punch" from life, stop your mind and do the following:

1. Ask, what's the worst that can possibly happen?
2. Prepare to accept it if you have to.
3. Proceed calmly to improve upon the worst.

Simple, yes, but certainly not easy.

Whether you have minutes, hours, days, months, or years to prepare for any traumatic event, suppressed emotions are a major cause of disease and premature death. Understanding the coping process will help you come out on the "other side" of it less jaded. In her book, *Death and Dying*, Elisabeth Kübler-Ross tells us to allow ourselves to move through five stages of coping as a natural course: Denial, Anger, Bargaining, Depression, and Acceptance.

As an example, let's apply these five stages to a traumatic event most all of us have experienced: The Dead Battery! You're going to be late to work, so you rush out to your car, place the key in the ignition, and turn it on. You hear nothing but a grind: The battery is dead.

Denial: What's the first thing you do? You try to start it again! And again. You may check to make sure the radio, heater, lights, etc. are off and then...try again.

Anger: "%$@^##& car!...I should have junked you years ago." Did you slam your hand on the steering wheel? I have. "I should just leave you out in the rain and let you rust."

Bargaining (realizing that you're going to be late for work): "Oh, please car, if you will just start one more time, I promise I'll buy you a brand new battery, get a tune up, new tires, belts and hoses, and keep you in perfect working condition."

Depression: "Oh God, what am I going to do? I'm going to be late for work. I give up. My job is at risk, and I don't really care any more. What's the use?"

Acceptance: "Okay. It's dead. Guess I had better call the auto club or find another way to work. Time to get on with my day; I'll deal with this later."

This is not a trivial example. In fact, we all go through this process numerous times a day. A dead battery, the loss of a parking space, a wrong number, the loss of a pet, a job, a move to another city, an overdrawn bank account, etc.

Things to remember are:

♣ Any *change of circumstance* can cause us to go through this process.

♣ We don't have to go through the stages in sequence. We can skip a stage or go through two or three simultaneously.

♣ We can go through them in different time phases. The dead battery could take maybe five to ten minutes, the loss of a parking space five to ten seconds. A traumatic event involving the Criminal Justice System can take years.

♣ The intensity and duration of the reaction depends on how significant the change-produced loss is perceived.

It was mentioned above that grieving only begins where the five stages of grief leave off. Grief professionals often use the concept of "grief work" to help the bereaved through grief resolution. A psychologist friend of mine shared that one common definition of grief work is summarized by the acronym TEAR:

T = To accept the reality of the loss
E = Experience the pain of the loss
A = Adjust to the new environment without the lost person or object
R = Reinvest in the new reality

Personally, I have found that "grief work" begins when the honeymoon period of the loss is over. That's the time when the friends have stopped calling, everyone thinks you should be over it, the court case is resolved, "closure" has been affected, and everything is supposed to be back to normal. Don't be surprised to find that this is the point that your real grieving begins. Don't pretend that it doesn't exist and "tough it out." This only delays your freedom from the searing pain of loss. Keep revisiting the cycle above and call upon the help of a counselor to guide you through these steps to their completion.

"The mind is its own place, and in itself can make a Heaven of Hell, a Hell of Heaven."
—John Milton

Stressorcise #10:
Overcoming Delegation Deficiency

So many of us have a hard time saying no to the requests of others. Perhaps we are afraid of hurting their feelings. Keep in mind, however, that each time you say yes to one thing, you say no to something else. Sometimes, saying no is best. Here is a simple but powerful way to "share the load" when everyone and everything seems to be competing for your time and attention.

Create a list all the activities that occupy your day, such as phone calls, meetings, major and minor projects, tasks for yourself, family, business/career/work and community—even the pets.

Choose from your list the three things that support your top three priorities in life. For example, if family, God, and work are your top three priorities in life, select which activities support these areas. This will be your focus and what I call your "high life value" activities.

Create a plan for delegating the rest of the activities on your list. This gives you more time, money, and energy to focus on what is really important to you. For example, hire a helper for around the yard or house to make more time available for family. It's kind of like having an assistant who gives you back the time lost by being busy with "stuff" instead of "invested" in your relationships.

Many boomers are doing everything else but what is important to *them*. Creating and keeping balance in your life requires that you sort through the pile of demands on your time and build greater balance between home, work, and recreation.

Stressorcise #11: Cell Phones and Email... Give It a Rest

The technology boom was supposed to make our lives easier and bring us closer. But has it? Answering email has gone from a task that takes a minute to one that could take hours. And our wireless tools keep beeping us and vibrating for us to "pick up, now!"

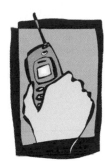

The problem lies in the fact that the instant communication boom has created the expectation for an instant response. Giving your cell number or email out to others implies that they may make instant demands on you.

In frustration, a friend recently shared with me how he feels about his wireless tools... "They're almost like an out-of-control paparazzi, zapping our ability to focus, draining our energy, and destroying our personal privacy.... And if left to their own devices (no pun intended) their constant interruptions can actually 'dis-empower' us more than they empowers us!"

Our ability to get in touch "instantly," anytime, anywhere, has become a non-stop intrusion into our world—and can cause a major drain on your body's battery.

Here's how to avoid information overload and be comfortable putting your cell phone and email on hold to buy back and enjoy some "quiet time."

- ❧ Shut it off while in restaurants, stores, the post office, meetings, etc.
- ❧ If your job or business has an "always available" policy, make it a habit to delegate some of the calls and e-responses to others according to the guidelines you give them.

♠ Set aside some "face time" to catch up with others, instead of multiple electronic "updates" throughout the day or week.

Create strong boundaries on your access by:

♠ Setting specific times that are off-limits for handling business or projects

♠ Taking yourself off others' general distribution lists

♠ Be honest about your availability when others call and ask, "Can you talk?"

Sure, you will still have a cell phone and email. However, you'll find that you have more time and control over your life if you don't constantly have to react to all the immediate needs of others.

If this feels uncomfortable, realize you only have so many hours in a day and that few people can get upset with you for keeping family a top commitment. Share with them that "It's nothing against you; it's just what I am doing for me to keep better balance between home and work."

Stressorcise #12:
Address the New Reality—
Caregiver Stress

Caregiver stress is a daily fact of life for over thirteen million boomers caught in the middle between the struggle for caring for themselves and caring for parents who are aging or suffering from chronic medical conditions such as cancer, stroke, multiple sclerosis, dementia, Alzheimer's disease, etc. Caregiving often takes a great deal of time, effort, and work. Many caregivers struggle to balance care-giving with other responsibilities including full-time jobs and caring for children. Constant stress can lead to "burnout" and health problems for the caregiver. Caregivers may feel guilty, frustrated, and angry from time to time.

The role of caregiver can drain them emotionally, physically, and financially as they do everything from lifting, bathing dressing, cooking, paying bills, shopping, giving medication, and providing company or emotional support, etc. Are you your parents' keeper? The role reversal of kids parenting parents can be scary and draining. Taking time for your own enrichment is critical for any caregiver. Failing to take care of yourself reduces your ability dramatically to take care of others. It's just like the flight attendants tell us on any flight about oxygen masks: "If the person next to you needs assistance, put your mask on *first*, and then help them put on theirs."

Caregiver stress is multifaceted because:

- ☸ The person you're caring for may be too ill to know you or follow simple plans.
- ☸ The person may be abusive emotionally or physically.
- ☸ The person may not recognize the caregiver or give him or her thanks for the effort.

Respite care can be a good way to get a break (respite) from constant caregiving. If other caregivers aren't available to fill in for the main caregiver, respite care services may be available in the community.

As a caregiver, you can take steps to take care of your own health:

- Eat a healthy diet rich in fruits, vegetables, and whole grains and low in saturated fat. Ask your healthcare provider about taking a customized nutritional supplement as well.
- Try to get enough sleep and rest.
- Find time for some exercise most days of the week. Regular exercise can help reduce stress and improve your health in many ways.
- See your healthcare provider for a checkup. Talk to your provider about symptoms of depression or illness that you may be having. Get counseling if needed.
- Stay in touch with friends. Social activities can help keep you feeling connected and help with stress. Faith-based groups can offer support and help to caregivers.
- Find a support group for other caregivers in your situation (such as caring for a person with dementia). Many support groups are available online through the Internet.

Resources include:

Well Spouse Foundation—www.wellspouse.org

Children of Aging Parents—www.caps4caregivers.org

Eldercare Locator—www.eldercare.gov

National Family Caregivers Association— www.nfcacares.org

Aging Parents & Elder Care— www.aging-parents-and-elder-care.com

Put Together Your Action Plan

As you can see, stress is your body's reaction to your thoughts, environment, and lifestyle. The key is to have it help you grow and to live with more zest as opposed to destroying your joy and energy for life. Take time every week to revisit the following:

Here's What's Happening: Identify your sources: examine your perceptions, interpretations, habits, and environment.

Here's How It's Affecting Me: Become aware of how your body responds and the symptoms that show stress is taking its toll.

Here's What I Am Committed to Do About It: Develop practical solutions: better skills, habits, and activities to cope more effectively and minimize the strain or trauma to your body and mind:

- Re-shaping attitudes
- Physical relaxation: deep breathing, muscle relaxation
- Mental relaxation: visualization, yoga, meditation
- Social support system
- Make regular deposits in the "emotional bank accounts" of yourself and other—keep your "I love yous" up to date. You never know when you may need to make a withdrawal.
- Change in environment
- Self-management related to time issues
- Proper nutrition
- Active exercise

For example, your action plan could look like this:

- ♠ To expand my social life and improve my social skills, I will _____.
- ♠ To begin nurturing and deepening relationships important to me, I will _____.
- ♠ To become more aware of my tension level, I will _____.
- ♠ To rest and recreate _____ , I will _____.
- ♠ To begin acknowledging my emotions and worth, I will _____.

Step #3:
Pursue Your Passion–Dream Big

Were you brought up to believe that reaching beyond what you have is bad? Guess what? *Dreaming is a healthy and wonderful way to stay young!* You create your future *from your future* not your past. Be a dreamer. Rid yourself of self-limiting beliefs and pursue a new destiny. If you talk to most people and ask them what they want, they will tell you what they don't want. Don't limit your life to what you don't want. Stoke a fire inside to pursue what you *do* want. Dream big! Ask yourself "what's missing," and revisit your purpose. Reinvest your time, energy, and emotions into reinventing yourself with a life script that keeps you young at heart. The size of your vision determines the size of your life.

> "When I examined myself and my methods of thought I determined that the gift of fantasy has meant more to me than my talent for absorbing positive knowledge."
> —Albert Einstein

Get Aboard the *Dream Express*

With some groundwork, the right mental attitude, good physical health (we'll get to that!), and a strong team (even of one), you can bring your dream to life. You will feel a sense of freedom as your dream enlarges instead of just caving in to fear of failure because of your limits in the past.

Make an unconditional commitment to leave the comfort zone behind. Never run away from your dream again. Pursue and live your dream, and break through your comfort zone with the Dream Express life map below.

Launching Pad (What draws you?)

What are the talents, gifts, and desires that inspire you? Ask yourself, if I could do anything I wanted, even for free, what do I really love or wish I could do? How bad do you want it? For some you're a CEO who wants to be a teacher or a non-professional who wants to translate foreign language skills into becoming a personal tutor. For others it's taking that decorating or home repair skills to a new level. Whatever it is, no matter how inconsequential it may seem to others, it's not to you. It's your *dream!*

The first step to re-inventing yourself is to break free of your comfort zone. I tell my clients, "I haven't seen my comfort zone in so long, I don't even know where it is. But I sure love the adventures of life."

> **"Life isn't about finding yourself. Life is about creating yourself."**
> —Anonymous

Take twenty minutes to invest in a new future for yourself. Make a list of what you want and why. What passion or excitement does it ignite inside of you? Include what it helps you to enjoy, and feel how it adds to your sense of fulfillment. Forget about the "how will I do this" part for now. We'll get to that later. If you don't like the word "dream," call it your "life aspirations wish list" for now...with a time table and plan attached.

Think about how you could explore new possibilities. Think beyond your old way of seeing yourself. Stop settling for less than you want. Think about what you would love to accomplish, if you followed your heart and knew you could not fail. Don't be fooled into thinking your past is your potential. Put it on your "life's dream" agenda, and develop a list of "*who* I am," instead of "*what* I am."

And don't be afraid of reaching too high. If it were easy, it wouldn't be a dream...would it? When I was 117 pounds, wanting to be a champion bodybuilder, I needed to reach deep inside and find the courage to act on behalf of the dream in my head, not my current skinny reality. Each workout, for over four years, I held the image of what I wanted to accomplish until my outside world matched my inside world, and I won over ten titles.

If you find yourself feeling inadequate or fearful of the size of your dream, keep in mind the words of Napoleon Hill, author of the bestseller, *Think and Grow Rich*: "Whatever the mind can conceive, and believe, it can achieve."

Comfort Zone (What Fear Holds You Back?)

Your biggest struggle is the competition between what you want and need—your desire for comfort and safety and your need for approval from others. To break through to the "other side" of your dream means you must break through your comfort zone by focusing on the prize instead of the price! What's been holding you back?

Force yourself to do something that *feels* uncomfortable until it becomes easier. Become a "disappointment dodger" instead of an "old codger." *Put more power in your self talk....* Be mindful of and protect your self talk.... Your mind has the ability to integrate or disintegrate your thoughts and continually build or slowly erode your inner wealth. In his bestseller, *Jonathan Livingston Seagull*, Richard Bach told us: "Sooner or later, those who win are those who think they can."

> **"We have met the enemy, and he is us!"**
> —Pogo

Boundary Zone

Realize that other people's boundaries and comfort zone may overlap yours and hold you back. They may not like that you are "venturing out" to go beyond their own limits and fears. If you find others threatened by your new plans, remember that each of us has the power to live the life of our dreams—or be limited by the fears of others.

I think that Jack Canfield (*Chicken Soup for the Soul*) puts it all into perspective best: "I like Dr. Daniel Amen's 18/40/60 rule: When you're 18, you worry about what everybody is thinking of you; when you're 40, you don't give a darn what anybody thinks of you; when you're 60, you realize that nobody's been thinking about you at all."

A good example of the boundary bashers include "do-gooders", who say things to you like: "After all I've done for you, why would you want to ___"...to the other end of, "It's okay, don't push yourself; we'll take care of you...." When you give away your ability to decide for yourself, you give up your ability to be yourself.

At the boundary zone you must decide what you want and go for it...or be okay living someone else's dream. You must decide to live either your life or theirs—it's just that simple.

> "Kites rise highest against the wind— not with it."
> —Sir Winston Churchill

Wasteland

Called so because you may get stuck due to feeling that every effort and day is a waste of time, energy, and money. That's your wasteland. Overcome this quagmire by focusing on your reward and end point, not where you are stuck. Make a mental and physical list of why you want this dream—not why you can't have it. If it was easy and readily attainable, it would not be a dream, would it?

Even if you can't move forward, you can turn right or left and keep moving. Sometimes it will be like driving though the fog. But if you keep moving, more of the road to your dream will appear. Instead of getting upset when things don't go as anticipated, always ask yourself, "What's the opportunity in this...what's the miracle in the madness?" If you hang in there, you will enjoy your dream!

A friend of mine once told me to keep in mind the power of one single thought: "If you think you can...or you think you can't...you're right."

> "If the dream is big enough the facts don't count."
> —Dexter Yager

Border Crossing—the Crossroads

You'll know you're at a crossroad when you stop and say, "Where do I go from here?...Which road do I choose?"

At the crossroads you have two choices: settle for what you have or focus on your dream and drive forward to experience something new. Become an inverse paranoid and expect the best at this stage. Instead of asking, "Why is this happening to me?" with feelings of disdain and the anticipation of possible failure...ask yourself instead, "What's the opportunity in this?... How is the world out to do me good, and what is it ready to bring to me?"

You have to want your dream bad enough to break through the barriers found at these crossroads. Some of our barriers could be time, what others think, health, finances, or fear of the unknown. Your courage must grow with your determination to live your dream. Courage is not attained without fear.... It's breaking through fear with positive self-action when you are confronted with obstacles and resistance. When you are at the crossroads, focus on your dream, commit to a direction, and do whatever it takes to get there.

Monster under the Bed

Remember when you were a kid and were afraid of the monster in the closet or under 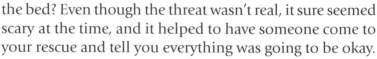 the bed? Even though the threat wasn't real, it sure seemed scary at the time, and it helped to have someone come to your rescue and tell you everything was going to be okay.

In order to get from where you are to where you want to be will require that you protect yourself from false fears generated by the influence of dream killers—the opinions of others. Like monsters under the bed, these dream killers seek out ways to influence and discourage you from changing the direction of your life. Keep in mind: This is your life, not theirs. To inoculate yourself from the mental pollution of others, make a list of dream supporters to serve as reality guides that will encourage and motivate you to aspire to new greatness. Use their energy to fuel yours as opposed to the toxic comments of others that drain you.

> **"Your focus determines your future."**
> —Brian Tracy

You will need to fall back on the support of yourself and others and spring forward with your vision and dream team.

Looking to write a book? One supporter may be a journalist or editor. Looking to get a new degree? Get the help of a professor who believes there is wisdom in aging.

Dreamland

Congratulations!! You are finally in a place to do what you've always wanted to do. But don't limit your dream now. All of this new "land" is your new comfort zone. The dream is never where you *are*. Our ever-expanding capacity expands as fulfillment grows. Make a list of new possibilities, and launch another life adventure.

There are no endings…only a series of new beginnings.

Remember Walt Disney did not stop at Disneyland. He went on to create Disney World and Epcot Center. Keep the *dream* alive, and you'll keep yourself alive!

> **"This time like all times is a very good one if we but know what to do with it."**
> —Ralph Waldo Emerson

Now What?

Putting it all together starts with a solid base. Reinvent yourself, and build your dream with these foundational questions. To give a broad, balanced coverage of all important areas in your life, ask yourself "What's missing?" in the following areas, and set some new goals:

Artistic:

Do you want to achieve any artistic goals? If so, what?

Attitude:

Is any part of your mindset holding you back? Is there any part of the way that you behave that upsets you? If so, set a goal to improve your behavior, or find a solution to the problem.

Career:

What level do you want to reach in your career?

Education:

Is there any knowledge you want to acquire in particular? What information and skills will you need to achieve other goals?

Family:

Do you want to be a parent? If so, how are you going to be a good parent? How do you want to be seen by a partner or by members of your extended family?

Financial:

How much do you want to earn by what stage?

Physical:

Are there any athletic goals you want to achieve, or do you want good health deep into old age? What steps are you going to take to achieve this?

Pleasure:

How do you want to enjoy yourself? You should ensure that some of your life is for you!

Public Service:

Do you want to make the world a better place by your existence? If so, how?

> "If we did all the things we are capable of doing, we would literally astound ourselves."
>
> —Thomas A. Edison

Step #4:
Find or Re-Define Passion in Your Work

If We're Going to Live Longer, What Are We Going to Do?

Webster's Dictionary defines retirement as: "dispose of," "to go away," "withdraw"… none of which describes an anti-aging boomer persona. In fact, a recent boomer study by AARP for the fifty years and older crowd found that eighty percent of those born between 1946 and 1964 plan to work into their retirement. However, it's not all about the money. According to longevity researcher Dr. Ken Dychtwald, the number one choice for the new boomer work ethic is a desire for a balance between work and leisure—not just the benefits and paycheck.

> "Your aspirations are your possibilities."
>
> —Dr. Samuel Johnson

The New Rx for Success?

According to the research of American Academy of Anti-Aging Medicine (A4M), a 2005 study by Merrill Lynch found that over 77 percent of men and women ages 40 to 58 plan to work in retirement. Part of making this a smooth transition—for *you*—begins by you being open to rediscover yourself. Discover your next calling.

What are you seeking? A new career? Championing some cause? Perhaps you need to rediscover or forge new vital relationships…with your spouse, kids, close friend, or new friends. Take advantage of some common resources (community groups, associates, or acquaintances) and revisit your purpose and reinvest your time, energy, and emotions into reinventing yourself and life script to stay young at heart—based on what matters most to you.

Reflecting on your personal stockpile of knowledge and experiences gives you an understanding of what you most enjoy and value and what types of learning experiences in the past have been most rewarding.

My mentor calls it "accomplishment feedback"… where you build on small wins and remind yourself not only of the risks but the rewards in store as well.

In his book *The Power Years*, Dr. Dychtwald shares that your rediscovery comes down to a couple of things:

- Envision what you want.
- Write it down as a vision statement.
- Act.

But he also shares that there are four boomer mindsets that influence our inspiration (inside force) and motivation (outside ourselves) to change.…which describes you?

- Ageless Explorers
- Comfortable Contents
- Live for Today
- Sick and Tired

Jet Fuel for Your Future
Adopt a New Mindset...
The World Is Your Classroom

In 2006 aging researchers claim that *every seven seconds a boomer in America turns fifty*. With this in mind, you may need to:

- Experience the joy of being a student again.
- Discover untapped interests.
- Hone your skills and give up your excuses.
- Satisfy your thirst for knowledge and self-mastery through independent study.

Create a personal master plan that outlines what life looks like if you have it better on your own terms:

- To begin taking charge of ____, I will ____.
- To expand my knowledge/personal power, I will read ____ pages or minutes a day in the areas of ____.
- To give back to others, I will ____.
- To gain a stronger spiritual sense and connection, I will ____.
- To begin seeing more of the good in life and others, I will begin to ____.
- Seek to deepen mentor and spiritual relationships by ____.

Should I Stay or Should I Go— Make Your Move

Aside from financial rewards or risks of moving, consider how and where you'll remake your life: Will you downsize or upsize? Will you relocate or revamp where you live? If a move is in the works for you, consider your preferences in the following to ensure optimal value and satisfaction with your move:

- Theme communities?
- Build your own?
- High rise?
- Pets, no pets?
- Alternative or traditional lifestyles?
- Religious or sexuality preferences?
- Kids?

Also, keep in mind what type of leisure or recreational setting is important to you:

- Group?
- Solitude?
- Nature?
- Efficiency Living or Elaborate?

In these modern nomadic times, I moved twelve times in ten years. Needless to say, I am not very fond of the smell of cardboard boxes, packing tape, or diesel fuel from moving vans. To minimize the stress of your move, research which city best fits your dreams, financial goals, beliefs, and personal values.

Career Change...Me? Now?

In the last thirty years my wife and I have had multiple career paths before arriving at our present place in life. There are three strategies to consider if you want to make a change without jeopardizing your finances:

1. Remain with your current employer but ask for flexibility in your role and hours to fit your goals and desired lifestyle better. Customize your job with unpaid leaves of absence; be available for temporary project management, etc. The objective here is to utilize your skills without wearing yourself out in the process.

2. Go to a new employer to pursue your passion in a different setting. Jumpstart this option by taking out a legal pad and making a list of the following:

- What do you value most?
- What is your greatest value to your employer?
- List how other businesses could use your mindset, skill set, and work ethic so that both of you get what you lack.
- Start your own business around things you value and enjoy.

3. After losing a job or career some boomers opt to invest themselves in their own business so they can integrate their passion with their paycheck. After losing his twenty-five-plus-year career with a major Detroit auto maker, Jerry decided it was time to have more control over his own destiny. After taking a few months off to regroup, research, and rebuild after his loss, he opened up a computer repair store to combine his passion with his pay.

Let's see how this would play out. Keep in mind that it can be not only challenging (which is not bad) but also a risk. You may or may not have time to rebuild your assets if the venture flops.

Research shows that the *top three risks of business ownership* are:

- Time deficiency
- Money deficiency
- Lack of balance between home and work life

Overcome these risks and enjoy the rewards by:

- Having a mentor who "knows the ropes"
- Having a plan
- Staying focused

I was able to rise from the "death" of a business failure doing the same. Be sure to lay a solid foundation, and remember that it is never too soon to start…draw on all resources at your disposal.

Making Your Encore a Reality…

Your new career is about much more that earning a living… It's an opportunity to shed your old life and to become exactly who you want to be by working at what you enjoy…and better yet, on your own terms. Regardless of how you choose to reinvent yourself, keep in mind it's the can-do attitude with which you approach anything—at *any* age—that makes a difference.

> "Nothing happens unless first a dream."
>
> —Carl Sandburg

- Follow these tips but also consult websites like www. 2young2retire.com …and www.retiredbrains.com.
- Build a team of support, and learn from the experience of others.
- Don't try to go it alone.
- Lean on a social network to introduce you to colleagues, friends, and family.
- Hire a business coach. My mom used to say, "Many hands make light of the work."
- While putting together your team, create a timetable with a strategy and the tactics to implement and by whom.
- List your goals, both immediate and long-term. As you look at the steps to get there, look at the gap in

your resources, and acquire the help you need to get there.

❧ Share your plan with mentors, and take action.

Whether you decide to focus your energies on a new job, employer, or business, keep in mind that you increase your worth by increasing your value. The key to becoming more valuable is continuous self-improvement. Get better at solving problems or providing new services for unmet need. A friend of mine started a designated driver service to give those who overindulge a safe ride home. For a modest fee, he picks them up and arranges for their cars to follow them home. Never stop seeking out ways to increase your value. This may require that you get more training, develop new skills, or create new relationships. Keep in mind, however, that the responsibility for getting better at what you do and how you do it is yours.

> "Everyone who got where they are had to begin where they were."
> —Richard P. Evans, author of
> *The Christmas Box*

Baby Boomer Life Detour... Straight Ahead

As you live your life, even as you read this book, you will uncover new opportunities to make changes. Some will be modest, while others may totally redefine who you are and what you want to do with the rest of your life.

Meet Dr. Catherine Dungan-McPhail, a fellow boomer filled with purpose, passion, vision, and courage. After thirty years in practice, she has decided to make a major detour—to refocus her practice on wellness care instead of the conventional sick care. As logical as it sounds, help-ing people stay healthy to prevent illness is no small feat. It will require her to focus her time, money, and energy into a new vision. And why would someone do this? Let's let her tell you:

I believe I can make a bigger difference, Tim, in my world. In the last thirty years in practice, I realize that I have always had a passion to help others to not just get through each day, but really maximize their life experience through greater personal wellness. I now see a way—filled with integrity, which addresses how to provide this service. I see a new way to provide all levels of health—physical, emotional, and biological. My true joy comes from living my purpose one hun-dred percent, and I want to help change the wellness of people in my community. I want to thank you for helping me to think differently.

Go to our web site (www.abetterboomerlife.com)
for information on her creating wellness program.

Now What? Putting It All Together

What you think about, talk about, and do something about usually comes about. What's your purpose and passion? Is it time for a detour? What needs to change? As you explore new possibilities, realize that you won't be starting from scratch. The things you have experienced and learned over a lifetime provide the blueprint for what you can live and learn as you move forward.

There are no "perfect" ideas, so just start somewhere.

> **"I believe the only reason we're here is to find out what we love...and get about the business of living it!"**
> —Oprah Winfrey

Step #5:
Mind Your Own Mind—Boost Your Brain Power

Losing your memory, becoming moody, or losing your "smarts" are not inevitable with aging.

In *The Better Brain Book* Dr. David Perlmutter, board certified neurologist, says, " by age 40, about two-thirds of all people experience some mental decline." However, he also points out: "When it comes to impaired brain function, age alone is not the primary culprit. Simply growing older doesn't mean that you will grow frail in body and mind."

There's a lot you can do to age-proof your mind and preserve its power before your next birthday. For starters, look at your life habits. Chronic stress, lack of sleep, and food additives can drain your brain, as can the regular use of prescription and over-the-counter medications.

What's in your medicine cabinet? A lot of the things we take to feel better in the short-term can affect our brain power in the long term. Antacids, birth control pills, certain pain relievers, and cholesterol-lowering drugs can all steal key nutrients (such as B vitamins, anti-oxidants, etc.) your brain needs for peak performance and to protect against disease.

Food for thought—what's on your plate? What you eat today has a major influence on what you get out of your brain tomorrow. MSG, sugar, artificial sweeteners, and a diet of more meat than vegetables can contribute to sub-par brain power.

Brain Fuel

Nutrition is key for optimizing your brain fuel. Nutritional supplements to boost brain power include:

- B vitamins from leafy greens and other things.
- Alpha-Lipoic Acid (ALA): a versatile antioxidant used to treat many age-related diseases, from stroke, diabetes, and heart attack to cataracts. It works by deactivating a host of cell-damaging free radicals.
- Fish Oil (EPA/DHA): works by protecting the brain against cell damage.
- Phosphatidylserine (PS): a phospholipid (a type of fat) that is found in every cell in the body. It helps increase communication across brain cells as you age—to keep you sharp, focused, and alert.
- Ginko Biloba: an antioxidant that helps protect brain cells from damage and increases circulation to the brain.

In his book *The Healing Nutrients Within*, Eric R. Braverman, M.D., explains how to use amino acids to fight Alzheimer's disease, depression, and other unhealthy aging issues. Another great reference is *The Brainpower Plan* by Jordan Davis, M.D. He reminds us that what's good for the heart is also good for the brain. The habits that prevent heart disease, diabetes, and stroke—such as anti-oxidants and exercise—can also protect your brain's health.

Other lifestyle factors that can strain or drain the brain include:

- Tobacco use
- Recreational drugs, such as cocaine
- Well water
- Inactivity
- Pesticides
- Lack of recreation
- Excessive alcohol consumption

Use It or Lose It: Plan for Mental Stimulation as Part of Your Day

According to memory expert Bill Beckwith (January 2006 *AARP Bulletin*), if you spend your time watching reality shows and reading the latest tabloid, you're headed for disaster—mentally speaking. To improve your mental capacity, he suggests that you:

> Stretch your brain, continue learning, expose yourself to new experiences. These can be as minor as taking a new route to work every day and as major as returning to school for another degree. As simple as completing the daily crossword puzzle and as complex as learning a new language.

Other Good Exercises for Strengthening Your Memory and Mental Flexibility

According to anti-aging experts from A4M (American Academy of Anti-Aging Medicine) and others:

- Don't use your calculator.
- Learn from books on tape.
- Don't use a shopping list; create a system to remember what you need.
- Vary your routine—brush your teeth with the opposite hand; put your clothes on in a different order.

Other brain-boosting exercises include learning to read upside down, memorizing poetry, and playing board games that stimulate your logic.

Remember This

Get in the habit of using your self-talk to get more of what you want to achieve, *not* what you want to avoid. Here is a simple way to get more, by forgetting less, using your keys as an example:

Instead of saying, "don't forget my keys," say "remember my keys." Although it may sound silly, it really works. If you talk to any golfers, they will agree by telling you how they have been using this positive self-talk principle successfully for years by saying to themselves "aim for the pin," as opposed to "avoid the sand trap or water."

Start the habit of focusing on what you want to *attain*, not on what you want to *avoid*. Replace "don't forget…" with one simple word, *remember*—and see what a difference it makes in your results.

> "My brain is my second favorite organ."
>
> —Woody Allen

Now What? Putting It All Together

Living a healthy life through balanced nutrition, regular exercise, and modifying your lifestyle can enable you to keep on top of your game—longer.

It is important to stimulate your memory and other mental functions by going back to the basics of reading, writing, and arithmetic, having an active social life and a positive outlook.

Be mindful of which lifestyle risk factors you may have for cardiovascular disease, and see your health professional for ways to decrease unnecessary medications.

Step #6:
Don't Wear Out Your Body

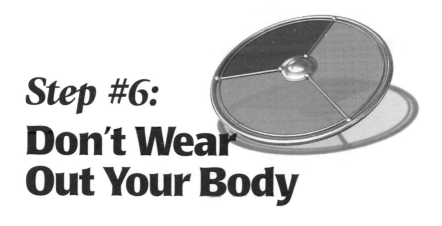

We are living longer than ever before. As a result, the consequences of what we do to our bodies will impact the quality of our lives as we age. Most baby boomers are clueless about how to keep our bodies from wearing out prematurely. Here are some simple, easy-to-implement solutions for putting some more sand back into the hour glass.

Restorative Sleep: How Much Is Your Night Stealing from Your Day?

When was the last time you had a good night's sleep? The fatigue you feel right now could be the result of the sleep you lost last night.

Restorative sleep is a major building block in the defense against aging. According to the National Sleep Foundation's 2002 Sleep in America Poll, 58 percent of adults in the U.S. experience insomnia. As a result, more and more doctors are finding that we're just not getting the restful sleep we need and are experiencing a variety of undesirable side effects, which can include:

- ♠ Lack of energy
- ♠ Depression

- ♨ Anxiety
- ♨ Poor memory
- ♨ Difficulty concentrating

When you fall asleep and remain asleep, your body is able to rebuild your energy and repair all cells that keep you at your best. If you experience trouble falling asleep or staying asleep, consider that aside from the dozens of prescription and non-prescription drugs known to sometimes interfere with normal rest, lifestyle factors such as caffeine, nicotine, and rigorous exercise before going to bed may be the culprit.

Do you forgo sleep to make room for work or leisure? You are not alone. Experts claim that regularly catching only a few hours of sleep can hinder metabolism and hormone production in a way that is similar to the effects of aging and early stages of diabetes. Chronic sleep loss may speed the onset or increase the severity of age-related conditions such as type 2 diabetes, high blood pressure, obesity, and memory loss.

New studies even suggest a link between sleep deprivation and an increased susceptibility to viral infection and a compromised immune system. Other studies have shown a link between sleep deprivation and bipolar disorder.

Lack of restorative sleep is an incredible disruption of our finely balanced hormones. Seven hours is an absolute minimum for almost all of us, and most of us would benefit from closer to eight hours.

The good news is that sleep debt can be made up. Spending more than the normal eight hours in bed can actually return the body's chemical balance to normal.

What's your bedtime? Studies indicate that the ideal time for you to go to bed is 10:00 P.M. During the winter months, perhaps 9:30 P.M. is best, especially if you awake early for work. You will find that you are more refreshed as an early-to-bed, early-to-rise person.

Sleep Disorders and You

If you have *sleep apnea*, you probably snore. Chances are good that snoring disrupts restorative sleep. Losing weight may help people with sleep apnea. It also helps to sleep on your side and to avoid alcohol and sleep medications. Surgery involving the nasal passageways (or uvula) may be an option in the event of an obstructive airway. Many people find relief with a nasal mask that keeps their air passage open during the night, the nasal Continuous Positive Airway Pressure (CPAP). Consult your doctor to see which option is right for you.

If you have *restless leg syndrome*, the frequent impulse to move your legs around (or even walk), especially at night, it may interfere with your ability to fall asleep and/ or your ability to obtain sound restorative sleep. Try placing hot or cold packs on your legs or taking a hot or cold bath for relief from the symptoms. Relaxation techniques noted in this book may help, too. You can also try massaging your legs, feet, and toes before going to bed. Consult your doctor to see which nutrients (such as magnesium) or sleep therapy is appropriate for your situation.

If you suffer from *periodic leg syndrome*, you find sleep to be elusive because of the unconscious movement (kicking) of one or both legs many times during the night. Consult your doctor for the appropriate therapy to reduce or eliminate your symptoms.

Here are some behavioral changes to foil the sleep stealers and increase the repair and revitalization of vital cells, organs, and tissues:

- ☀ Get a new mattress: make your bed your haven instead of a hindrance for sleep.

- Set a sleep schedule: go to bed and get up at the same time every day.
- Limit naps to twenty minutes or less.
- Avoid caffeine after lunch.
- Don't drink alcohol in the evening.
- Don't drink anything within two hours of going to bed.
- Take a hot shower, bath, or sauna before going to bed.
- Remove the clock from view.
- Keep your bed a place for sleeping—not working or watching television.
- Don't lie in bed for more than thirty minutes to go to sleep. Get up and do something quiet for a while (reading or listening to music)…then try again to fall asleep.
- Ask your doctor if your medications could be a problem with sleep.
- Consult your doctor if allergies, pain, or discomfort rob you of your sleep.
- Exercise earlier in the day to melt away the stored stress of the day.
- Keep your bedroom temperature between sixty-five and seventy degrees.
- Lose weight.
- Reduce the number of medications (prescription and over-the-counter) that you are taking.

  If the behavioral changes don't help, consider these other options:
- Increase your melatonin levels. Try to expose yourself to more natural, bright sunlight during the daytime; use full spectrum fluorescent bulbs in the winter and sleep in complete darkness at night. You

can even eat a high-protein snack several hours before bed to increase your body's melatonin and
serotonin levels.

● Have your adrenals checked by a good natural medicine clinician. Scientists have found that insomnia
may be linked to adrenal stress.

● If you are menopausal or peri-menopausal, get
checked out by a good natural medicine physician.

> **"A wise healer uses all that works."**
> —Dr. Mark Houston

Now What?

For more information on minimizing the wear and
tear on your body, visit www.mercola.com or www.
familydoctor.org.

Other areas to include are your nutritional and exercise habits, which are covered next.

Step #7:
The Impact of Nutrition on a Vibrant Life

Let's keep it simple. Eating is something we all do, but too often we make the wrong choices. Living longer and better doesn't require extreme diets or lifestyles. The focus here is not to tell you what to give up—anyone can do that—but what you can *take up* to boost your "nutritional bank account." Like your checkbook, your body must maintain a positive balance of nutrients to cover the nutritional debt of your lifestyle and habits. For example, people who smoke or have high-stress lifestyles require higher amounts of B and C vitamins, as well as certain minerals and amino acids.

An anti-aging lifestyle is based on the premise that many of the chronic (long-term) diseases associated with aging—hypertension, cardiovascular disease (CVD), diabetes, osteoarthritis, and osteoporosis—are not an inevitable outcome of aging. Instead, to a large extent, these diseases are preventable simply by making smarter nutritional choices. Things that many people view as signs of aging—such as low energy, poor memory, low libido, chronic pain, and weight gain—often are not signs of aging at all. They are signs of inadequate nutrition and lifestyle management.

Anti-Aging from the Inside Out

Adopting a few healthy nutritional habits can delay the onset of illnesses considered to be a part of "old age" and increase your years of optimal health and life enjoyment. Here's how. Number one…give food the attention it deserves. Focus on three key areas to optimize your nutritional power:

1. The frequency of what you eat
2. The amount that you eat
3. The type of food you eat

Putting it into practice is as simple as:

- Make time to eat meals every three to four hours. Skipping meals allows hunger to build, causing you to overeat when you finally get to eat again.
- Avoid eating within an hour of going to bed. A full stomach can keep you up.
- Limit beverages, especially cold beverages, to a cup or less per meal.
- Buy smaller dishes to reduce the amount you serve yourself.
- Eat off of plates, *not out of packages*.
- Whenever possible, eat in a quiet, relaxed atmosphere. Tense muscles (in your stomach) inhibit digestion.
- Chew your food well. It aids in digestion.
- Keep quick fixes around to munch on, such as dried fruits, nuts, and food bars for nutritional emergencies until full nutrition can be replenished. Read the label and choose varieties with the least sugar or sulfites.

The Value of an Old Friend

Remember when you were at a water park and saw the water slide. Imagine if there was little or no water… what would happen? Friction and even a total stop of momentum would result—causing the slide to back up and shut down. Your body needs water in the same way.

The Importance of Hydrating Yourself Properly

Water is the predominant compound in your body—about seventy-eight percent of your body weight at birth, dropping to about seventy-two percent of our fat free weight as we age. Water is a natural lubricant that helps everything run smoothly. When your body becomes low on water, it will pull fluids from your joints to keep your brain and heart afloat. If not corrected, however, orthopedic specialists tell us that this diversion can lead to joint degeneration and arthritis. According to the National Institute of Health and the Mayo Clinic, proper water intake is also vital for:

- Acting as a cushion to protect your organs
- Building moisture in your mouth, eyes, and nose
- Deterring bad breath
- Digestion
- Dissolving and aiding in the absorption of vital nutrients
- Enhancing mental clarity
- Excreting water-soluble waste through the urine
- Increasing energy
- Maintaining a healthy body weight
- Regulating your body's temperature
- Transporting vital nutrients and oxygen to your cells

As you can see, water supports all body processes. But don't rely on thirst alone to tell you when to drink more of this liquid gold. Thirst usually does not develop until after all your cells have been depleted and your body is running on empty. Nutrition experts suggest a half ounce of water for each pound of weight—the proverbial eight eight-ounce glasses a day. Keep in mind, however, that the following situations may increase your water needs:

- If you're taking diuretics
- If you're on a high protein diet
- If you have the flu or a cold
- If you engage in heavy physical activity or athletics
- If you live in an area with high temperature regions
- Dry winter air

Ignorance Is Not Bliss

Here are some signs and symptoms that show you may be "running on empty" and that water is a nutritional priority for you:

- Constipation
- Dry nose, mouth, or throat
- Dark, strong-smelling urine in small quantities
- Dry skin
- Fatigue and weakness
- Headaches
- Irritability
- Nausea
- Stomach cramps

As you can see, denying yourself optimal water supply accelerates the aging process because the water table of your body directly or indirectly participates in all biological functions. How much water did you drink so far today?

Flood Your Cells with the Good Stuff

We're talking H_2O, *not* soda pop, tea, coffee, juice, or the like. These can leave you tired, bloated, dehydrated, hungry, and fat. Other things that get in the way of you getting good water include the pipes that carry your water to your home and ground water quality of some wells. Many good water products and treatment systems are available to solve this dilemma and help you to nourish your body with water—just do your homework before selecting one. Finally, urologists claim that the main cause of most kidney stones is dehydration, so it is also essential to keep your body hydrated.

Health and Longevity Begin in the Gut!

When you consider all the things that go down your house's drain—razor stubble, soap scum, food, toilet paper, sand from the beach, and an occasional piece of jewelry—it becomes clear that plumbing can handle a lot. That's why we take steps to help clear the pipes, so things run smoothly.

It's the same with your body's pipes—your digestive system. Over the years we all put an extraordinary amount of things down our body's drain. We expect our plumbing to transport everything to the cells and down the tube to eliminate waste. When it doesn't, we experience digestive problems like clogs, spills, leaks, and a break in the lines—causing things like constipation, irritable bowel or "leaky gut" syndrome, etc.

Your intestines are living things—they're organs just like your heart and lungs. This extremely efficient system breaks down, absorbs and distributes the raw material you need to thrive, while eliminating the toxins produced by digestion and normal metabolism.

Ladies and Gentlemen, Start Your Digestive Engines—and Go!

When you consider that starch digestion begins in the mouth, you see the importance of keeping your teeth healthy through regular dental exams. Your ability to chew food thoroughly has a direct impact on the nutrition you gain from it. The act of chewing jumpstarts the release of enzymes needed by your stomach to extract the raw materials you need and satisfy "The Four Rs": rebuild, restore, repair, and revitalize all body systems.

A well cared for and lubricated system helps you live longer and better. Adequate water and fiber (as well as food supplements) help to ensure that this occurs. And speaking of fiber…fiber is not a nutrient, but it plays a key role in the optimal functioning of your digestive system and the maintenance of your internal plumbing. Found solely in plant food, it's the only part of plants that cannot be digested. Because most of us tend to eat too many processed foods, we miss out on a lot of fiber. Fiber is found in all vegetables and fruits, beans, seeds, and nuts.

What's the Big Deal?

Fiber helps keep things bulky and smooth as they move through our digestive system and eliminates built-up toxins and waste that can block the absorption of nutrients your body needs to function properly. Both soluble and insoluble fibers are good for you.

Soluble sources include: beans, barley, oats and oat bran, citrus fruits, peas, strawberries.

Insoluble sources include: apples, beets, Brussels sprouts, cabbage, carrots, brown rice, whole wheat cereals.

Be careful of the store-bought agents as they can have extra sweeteners and bulking agents added that may affect you adversely.

In real age years, people who eat twenty-five grams of fiber a day can be as many as three years younger than those who eat only twelve grams (the average for most adults). Adding fiber to your diet is a simple lifestyle change with huge rewards.

In his most recent book, *You: The Owner's Manual*, longevity expert Dr. Michael F. Roizen shares that a ten gram increase in daily fiber intake decreases the risk of heart attack by 29 percent—and makes you 1.9 percent years younger! Here are some of his top picks for quick fiber sources.

Quick Fiber Sources?

Lima Beans (3T)	=	13 grams
Buckwheat (1 cup)	=	10 grams
Artichoke (1 large)	=	10 grams
Soybeans (1/2 cup)	=	10 grams
Almonds (24)	=	5 grams
Peanuts (30)	=	5.5 grams
Oatmeal (1 cup)	=	3–4 grams

Experts also suggest that you supplement food with the power nutrients (covered later on).

What Does Cooking Have to Do with It—The Fresher the Better!

How you cook your food has everything to do with how much nutrition you get from it. Take a look at the impact various cooking methods have on the antioxidants (flavinoids) you gain from broccoli:

- ❧ Steamed: lost 11%
- ❧ Pressure cooked: lost 81%
- ❧ Micro-waved: lost 97%… This is a critical loss seeing as flavinoids are great anti-aging nutrients.

Other Nutrition Robbers

We live in a land of plenty and have a variety of foods at our fingertips. How is it that we eat more, yet get fewer nutrients? Unfortunately, most of our diets are comprised of more fats, sugars, and carbohydrates, with a void of nutritionally rich foods. In addition to these calorie- rich and nutritionally poor foods, many common aspects of daily living can deplete your body of the nutrients it needs to function properly.

Talk with your heath provider about how to reduce or avoid these common nutrient thieves:

- ❧ Alcohol
- ❧ Antacids
- ❧ Caffeine
- ❧ Nicotine
- ❧ Highly processed foods
- ❧ Prescription medications
- ❧ Over-the-counter medications
- ❧ Stress
- ❧ Illness

- Injury
- Hospitalization
- Intestinal problems
- Dieting

These things can rob vital nutrients from your system in three ways:

- They can increase the nutritional needs of your body (see below).
- They can accelerate the formation of free radicals and cause your body to lose nutrients.
- They can impair the absorption of nutrients from the food you eat.

As a result, they have the capacity to impact your health immensely. What can you do?

Don't Get Too Radical

Realize that a glass of wine here or a latté there won't destroy you. We are looking for balance in order to eliminate the excess formation of what science calls free radicals.

Free radicals are a group of chemicals that can cause damage to our cells, impairing our immune system, leading to various chronic and degenerative disorders. Similar to the browning effect of an apple or meat left out too long, free radicals age the body faster. Free radicals are normally kept in check by a nutritional group of aging avengers called antioxidants that neutralize them. Although normally manufactured in the body, research shows there is tremendous value in supplementing your diet with these nutritional vanguards for vitality.

Food Supplements: Hype or Hope?

Talk to your healthcare provider for the best nutritional weapons to supplement your diet in order to compensate for these situations that impact your body or cause nutritional losses. Their recommendations include the following *power nutrients as life extension boosters*:

- ❧ Omega-3, the healthy fat that helps prevent hardening of the arteries and other benefits
- ❧ Probiotics—the stomach's "friendly bacteria"
- ❧ Antioxidants—the vitamins, minerals, and enzymes that improve circulation and protect your cells from the formation of "free" radicals, such as: beta carotene (helps body make vitamin A), vitamin C and E, CoQ10, N-Acetyl Cysteine, selenium and other compounds from green tea or grape seed extract, etc.
- ❧ Water—filtered, not tap
- ❧ Fiber
- ❧ Specific minerals and amino acids
- ❧ *"P.S."—I love you.* They may also suggest phosphatidylserine (PS) to help improve brain power and keep you sharp.

Food as Your Friend

Make sure the food you eat provides more than calories alone. It must provide the raw materials from which your hair, skin, muscle, bone, and all other tissues are grown and sustained. Your diet provides the nutrients necessary to manufacture the enzymes and hormones that control the function of every cell in your body. Your body also uses these nutrients to make neurotransmitters that regulate how you think and feel. Needless to say, ensuring proper balance of macro-nutrients (protein, carbohydrates, and fat) and micro-nutrients (vitamins, minerals, and other food components) is key to the rate and way in which your body ages.

You really are what you eat. The benefits from eating healthy are endless. Many people know about the benefits of vitamins, but few know about the key role of minerals, which are the basic building blocks of connective tissue (bones, muscles, tendons, ligaments, discs, skin, etc.). Some superstar foods to help you age more gracefully include:

- ♠ Acai Fruit: This little berry is one of the most nutritious and powerful foods in the world. It can often be found in juice form in health food and gourmet stores.

- ♠ Anything in the "Allium Family"—garlic, onions, leeks, scallions, chives, and shallots all can help the liver eliminate toxins and carcinogens.

- ♠ Barley: This can be used as a breakfast cereal in soups and stews and as a rice substitute. Barley is also high in fiber, which helps metabolize fats, cholesterol, and carbohydrates.

- ♠ Green Foods: Green foods like wheat and barley grasses can be bought in powder, tablet, or juice form and offer greater levels of nutrients than green leafy vegetables. They also help to moderate cholesterol, blood pressure, and immune response.

- ♠ Buckwheat, Seed, and Grain: Buckwheat is loaded with protein, high in amino acid, aids in stabilizing blood sugar, and reduces hypertension.

- ♠ Beans and Lentils: You can reduce cholesterol while beefing up on antioxidants, folic acid, and potassium. Try kidney, black, navy, pinto, chickpeas, soybeans, peas, and lentils.

- ❧ Hot Peppers: Both bell and chili peppers contain antioxidants, have twice the Vitamin C as citrus fruit, and work great as fat burners.
- ❧ Nuts and Seeds: You can't go wrong with a handful of nuts a day—walnuts, hazelnuts, almonds, macadamia, and pistachio nuts contain Omega 3 fats, which are great for your heart. Raw, unsalted nuts and seeds are best. Flax seeds also add Omega 3 and six fatty acids. Adding a tablespoon of ground flax seeds a day to your cereal, soups, and salads is a great way to put more flavor, fiber, Omega 3 fats, and lignans (a plant compound that some scientist say boosts your immune system) into your diet.
- ❧ Sprouts: These "baby veggies" are grown from seed to salad in a week. Numerous varieties of sprouts are great with any meal. They're a great source of protein, phytochemical, and Vitamin C. By adding them to any dish your immune system will get a boost.
- ❧ Yogurt and Kefir: When you consider that over seventy percent of your immune system involves your digestive tract, these cultured foods make a lot of sense. They contain healthful bacteria that aid in digestion and building your immune function, as well as add calcium. Try using them as a base for a smoothie or salad dressing.

In *Blood Sugar Blues* Miryam Williamson emphasizes the tremendous impact nutrition has on your health: "There is no disease or disorder that cannot be made worse by poor diet. There is none that can't be improved by changes in lifestyle, especially where nutrition is concerned."

Keep in Mind the Diet/Insulin Connection

Insulin is a hormone that responds directly to what you eat. Two of its many roles are to regulate fat metabolism and control blood sugar. Blood sugar is the basic fuel that all cells in your body use to make energy. In optimal circumstances, the body maintains your blood sugar level. However, too much blood sugar leads to hyperglycemia. Maintaining the ideal range (not too low or high) is the key not only to energy but also your health.

Get Familiar with the Glycemic Index of Foods

Foods that produce high levels of blood sugar are called high glycemic index (GI) foods (see appendix). When your diet consists of a high amount of these foods, your body responds by producing higher levels of insulin than it would if you were eating lower GI foods. When insulin levels are high, your body not only converts blood sugar into energy, but also stores the extra energy as fat. So, when insulin levels are high, you store more fat. When insulin levels are low, you burn fat more efficiently and maintain a balance between blood sugar and insulin.

Additionally, a diet predominantly of high GI foods can lead to carbohydrate cravings and overall increase in appetite—potentially leading to increased fat weight. These foods can cause large fluctuations in blood sugar and insulin levels, leading to a vicious cycle of fatigue and overeating.

> "The platter kills more than the sword."
> —Sir William Osler

The Death of Diets

Most programs dealing with weight loss and weight control focus exclusively on taking away food. Considering that you will eat over one thousand meals this year, it doesn't make sense to limit forty or fifty of them (which is what you do when you go on a "diet") and hope to succeed at both weight loss and control.

Taking away food because you have a problem with your weight makes as much sense as taking away your paycheck because you have a problem with your finances. Success in each of these areas requires that you lose bad habits and gain better ones to get and keep more of what you want.

Dieting is a major nutritional thief. It not only limits essential nutrients for skin tone, hair color, and overall health, but it also encourages a loss of self-respect because of the unrealistic demands it places on you and your life!

A life of diets can also lead to bone and muscle loss, hypoglycemia, hair and skin disorders and loss of sex drive, not to mention the onset of degenerative type diseases that erode your quality of life—each of which will also impact your finances and self-esteem.

Just say *no* to dieting! There is more to losing weight and keeping it off than just giving up food. Identifying and modifying your nutrition, exercise, and attitude habits is the key to your long-term success. Meet with a wellness professional to evaluate your current health, set up a plan to lose excess body fat, and gain greater wellness and confidence. In the meantime, start replacing your diet habits with slender habits:

Start Your Day with Breakfast

Break-the-fast to gear your body for the day's demands. Then:

1. *Eat Smaller Meals*—Make it easier to digest and absorb full nutritional value. Fill up *not* out.

2. *Eat More Frequently*—Skipping meals can cause blood sugar crashes that lead to dizziness, hunger, or fatigue. If your ideal calorie intake is 1,700 calories a day, it is better to consume those calories in several (four to five) smaller meals than in three large ones. People who refuel their body on this type of schedule are very pleased that they are eating more and gaining less!

3. *Drink Half Your Body Weight in Ounces of Water (i.e., a one-hundred-pound person should drink fifty ounces of water)*—Not tea, coffee, juice, etc. Include at least one glass of water for every three hours you're awake.

4. *Eat Slowly*—Digestion begins in the mouth. The more you chew your food, the better your digestion before you leave the table, helping you avoid bloating, indigestion, or overeating.

5. *Snack Right*—Look for low-fat, low-sodium, low-sugar choices throughout the day.

Catch yourself in the act. It can be said that we live by our habits—especially when it comes to food. So often, we watch TV, work, or just go about our day without being aware of how much and how often we eat. Like everything else in life, awareness is our first line of defense for greater control. To see if your eating habits are helping or hindering your goals, fill out a "what I consume" log for the next seven days. You will be amazed at what it reveals.

The following story illustrates the point best: A university conducted a study in which twenty-five overweight students were asked to keep a faithful record of everything they ate or drank. After three weeks they turned in their food diaries and were placed in a dorm under the supervision of dieticians.

For the next three weeks they were fed exactly what they said they had eaten. And guess what? They lost an average of ten to fifteen pounds.

Be *fair* to yourself. *Never* exclude your favorite foods just for the sake of nutrition. A little chocolate, etc. won't hurt you—unless, of course, food allergies or other medical conditions require you abstain from eating them. It is the dominance of these foods in the past that made them a problem. You will find as you eat better that your cravings will diminish as well.

The Low-Fat Lie

Many people falsely believe that "low-fat" equals low calorie and better health. Although no one should be "fat phobic," the truth is…

When fat is removed from processed food, sugar is added in greater amounts to enhance flavor and taste. As a result, although fat is lower, sugar becomes a predominant ingredient. This increased amount of refined sugar (whether it is called sucrose, fructose, or something else) leads to high insulin secretion, which may lead to increased hunger, fat storage, and stress on the insulin balance mechanism in the body. It is kind of like "out of the frying pan and into the fire" from a nutritional standpoint (as discussed under "glycemic index of foods" later on in this section).

But I've Done All That

Losing weight can be easier or harder than you think. If you find that the excess fat just won't leave—no matter what you do—you may need more than a change in lifestyle to get things right. You could have underlying health issues (that you are not aware of) that make you gain weight or prevent you from losing it. Identifying your health issue and treating its cause can be in many cases very simple. Working with a physician trained and board certified in anti-aging medicine (see the "Doctor, Doctor" section of this book) can help your body regain the natural internal balance it needs for you to get and keep control over your weight.

Once your body's chemistry is optimized, you will find it easier to balance all lifestyle factors that affect your weight:

- When you eat...eat more often.
- How much you eat...eat less per sitting.
- Why you eat...no more swallowing your emotions.
- What you eat... more lean and green, more nutritional power, and fewer calories per serving.
- Replace calorie-storing activities with calorie-burning activities (more walking, hiking. swimming, aerobics, yoga, or palates...and *less* TV, computer, reading, sedentary crafts, etc.)—reminding you it's great to be alive!

A Final Word on Supplements

In *Nutritional Influences on Illness*, Melvyn R. Werbach presents overwhelming evidence confirming that nutritional deficiencies impact your health and quality of life—and even if you eat a balanced diet, your body can be deficient in the nutrients that are essential for optimal health. However, be sure you get as much out of the supplements you take as their manufacturers get out of you.

The new fifth edition of *The Nutrition Almanac* (Dunne, Lavon J., Dunne, Lavon) contains the latest scientific information on why, when, and how to supplement your diet for optimal benefit. It examines both the connections between nutrition and disease and custom nutrition regimes you can use to defend against or overcome the challenges and illnesses caused by deficiencies. Other excellent resources include *The Real Vitamin and Mineral Book* by Shari Lieberman, Ph.D., and *The Healing Nutrients Within* by Eric Braverman, M.D., who explains how to use amino acids to fight heart disease and more.

Now What? Putting It All Together

Make a list of the nutritional habits you can start to promote your longevity and quality of life. Align your health goals with the best FAT principle (Frequency, Amount, and Type of foods you eat) using a simple formula such as:

Choose more of these	Over these
fresh	leftovers, instant, or highly processed
low to medium glycemic high nutritional content	high glycemic empty calorie foods
filtered water	tap water, soft drinks, including diet
unsweetened juices	juices with added sweeteners
green tea/herbal teas	more than two to three cups coffee, including decaf
quick sauté, steamed prep	microwave, pan fired, deep fried
lean fish, fowl, meats, and vegetable oils	trans/hydrogenated/or saturated fats

Revamp your fridge and cupboards—add more foods that maximize your longevity and energy, and remove those things that accelerate your aging and erode your quality of life.

Be supermarket savvy—be prepared for "nutritional emergencies" with healthful snacks (low-sugar/ fat/ sodium types).

Become a menu master—whenever possible, select clear broth sauces and soups over cream varieties, more lean meat and veggies over pasta and cheese, baked over fried, more egg whites than yolks in your omelets, and mixed green salads over iceberg lettuce.

Boost your nutritional bank account utilizing a custom supplement plan to fill gaps in your nutritional needs.

Make time to eat in a more relaxed manner as opposed to "on the run." You are not only what you eat, you are what your body can absorb.

Don't become a slave to perfection—only consistency! Give your body the nutrients it needs to do the job you expect.

And remember…over seventy percent of your age-defying immune system is found in your digestive tract.

Step #8:
Get Physical, Baby—From the Inside Out!

Who's That in the Mirror?

Looking your best is an *inside out* process. You start with how you feel about yourself, continue with how you take care of yourself, and end with how you present yourself, on the outside. The person you see in the mirror is the person others see.

Do you look fresh and vibrant or dull and worn-out?

We can have confidence in our accomplishments, feel successful, have wonderful relationships and great families—and still not be happy about ourselves. Why?—because the person in the mirror is a stranger. How we think we look and how we actually look can be very different and very hard for many of us to accept. Our minds can be vibrant with energy, knowledge, and ideas—*we feel young*. We have goals to accomplish and a lot of living to enjoy. But…who is that person in the mirror? *We look old*. When did that happen?

Let's face the facts. Yes, we are older, and we deserve every wrinkle and gray hair we have; we worked hard for them. We just don't want to see them. Science has brought many avenues to alter our appearance to look younger.

This may or may not be an option for you. So…what can you do?

Because I think women have these thoughts more than men, here are some things to think about:

To Get Started, Try This Easy and Inexpensive Makeover

1. *When was the last time you changed your hair style?*
   - ❧ Replace dull gray hair…with a rich color.
   - ❧ Replace long lifeless strands…with a bouncy medium cut.
   - ❧ Replace the old frosted bob…with a sprouty short cut with highlights.

2. *When was the last time you changed your make-up?*
   - ❧ Replace the frosty robin-egg blue eyeshadow…with a matte mauve or soft brown/beige.
   - ❧ Replace the thick black eyeliner…with a soft kohl blue or brown.
   - ❧ Pluck eyebrows (they frame the picture of your face).
   - ❧ Use under eye concealer (to look well rested and accent your eye color).
   - ❧ Use a natural color foundation (for a flawless, even-toned complexion).
   - ❧ Use and apply a soft blush (to perk up cheeks for a pretty smile).
   - ❧ Use lip color and moisture (the final touch with pink tones to make teeth look whiter).

3. *Do you buy clothes to complement your best features?*
   - ❧ Look fresh and trendy, without being too "out there."

🌑 Shop with an honest friend who will tell you what looks better. She will tell you what compliments your figure or does not.

🌑 Hold up two colors (a warm peach and soft cool pink) by your face in front of the mirror and look carefully at your facial features. One will make you look older and tired, and one will make you look younger and awake. Which one suits you? Choose your wardrobe accordingly.

Now, look at the new and improved, graceful, fine, and beautiful person in the mirror. That's *you*...only better!

Energize with Exercise

If you take time to research the Industrial Revolution, it will show you that in 1830, thirty percent of the American economy was powered by muscle. In the last century that figure has withered to one percent or less.

As a result, today's fitness boom is actually a natural reaction to progress in America—and not just a passing fad. In order to maintain our bodies as well as our parents did, we must now plan for activity that was once part of a normal day. We no longer need to chop wood, scrub wooden floors, or hunt and harvest for our meals. Although progress is a good thing, we still need to replace the activities lost to labor-saving devices such as the lawn mover, washing machine, automobile, and others.

Exercise can help you change your family's health blueprint and roll back your body clock to enjoy better health and wellness for a lifetime. Take a look at how, over the years, our body makes changes in the following areas, all of which are improved through a personal fitness plan:

Variable	With Age	With Fitness
Strength	Decreases	Increases
Flexibility	Decreases	Increases
Stamina	Decreases	Increases
Bone Density	Decreases	Increases
Body Fat %	Increases	Decreases
Muscle Mass	Decreases	Increases

Experts claim that in addition to reducing health risks, exercise helps with decision- making and reducing pain. In *You: The Owner's Manual* Dr. Roizen shares studies showing that executives who participate in a regular exercise program make ten percent more income than those living a sedentary lifestyle. One study revealed that a sixty-year-old fit man actually has the function of a sedentary thirty-year-old.

Perhaps the most powerful tool in controlling the aging process and restoring vitality is to improve your muscle-to-fat ratio through exercise. In the last fifty years the amount of activity we get with daily chores has dropped four hundred calories per day. That's four hundred *fewer* calories we can consume before we can lose weight.

> "I joined a health club last year, spent about $300. Haven't lost a pound and don't feel any different. Apparently the gimmick is you have to show up."
> —Anonymous

What's the secret to the best exercise program for boomers? One that includes the balance and goals found with the FITT principle:

- ♠ *Frequency*: Fitness experts recommend exercising four times a week (check with your doctor first).
- ♠ *Intensity*: Get your heart rate up to at least 50% of its maximum capacity—ask your doctor about your number.
- ♠ *Time*: Usually forty-five minutes to an hour incorporating the three types below.
- ♠ *Type*: A balance of cardiovascular, resistance (body-sculpting and weights), and flexibility exercises.

Keep in Mind:	To Make It Last:
Warm up	Find something you like
Monitor intensity	Set a goal
Cool down	Make time
Stretch properly	Have an alternate plan
Have fun and make it a habit	Challenge yourself

Ask fit boomers, and they will tell you: "Anyone willing to invest three to four hours a week can enjoy the benefits of exercise." At eighty, a good friend of mine works out with her forty-plus-year-old son everyday on the weights.

She recently shared with me the results of her workouts: "Age has nothing to do with it…. It's lifestyle. I feel better at seventy-eight than I did at fifty."

Years ago, people in their fifties were recovering from heart attacks. Today, they're recovering from a good workout or exercise session, taking ballroom dancing and climbing mountains to reach new peaks of physical confidence and power. Keep in mind that jumping to conclusions and sidestepping responsibilities are not exercise.

> "The only reason I would take up jogging is so I could hear heavy breathing again."
> —Mark Houston, M.D.

The Fitness Advantage...Gaining the insight you need to set and reach goals you can *live with* by knowing your body composition.

Body Composition– The New Bathroom Scale

Is it possible to be overweight and in top shape or underweight and overly fat? You bet it is! One of the most 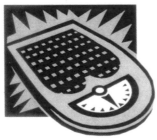 powerful changes you can make to reduce your risk of "growing old before your time" is to improve your body composition.

What is meant by body *composition*? Generally speaking, your body composition can be broken down into two parts: body fat and lean muscle mass. Body fat is just that—fat. Lean body mass includes everything in your body except fat (e.g., muscle, bones, organs, tissues, fluids, etc.). Although a certain amount of body fat is necessary (10–15% for men and 15–20% for women), a high fat-to-lean ratio is undesirable because it increases your health risks.

Healthy Body Composition Reduces These Health Risks for Diseases of Aging

- High blood pressure
- Low lean-to-fat body mass
- Abnormal cholesterol/metabolism
- Decreased muscle mass
- High insulin levels
- High triglyceride levels
- Decreased strength

You May Be Over-Fat Even If You're Not Overweight

According to the National Institute of Health, sixty percent of Americans are overweight—the highest number in history. But even if you are not overweight, you may have too little muscle and too much fat, a condition called *"sarcopenic obesity."* This medical term describes the age-related loss of muscle mass and function that adds to your health risk and accelerates the aging process.

A proper muscle-to-fat ratio has been associated with longevity and reduced risk of chronic disease. But you can't measure body composition by stepping on a scale. You measure it by using one of several devices usually available through your local gym or wellness center. Some manufacturers even make home use models available. Methods these devices can use include:

- Bioelectrical Impedance
- Skin-Fold Thickness
- Waist Circumference
- Infra-Red Light
- Hydrostatic Weighing
- Ultrasound Measurement

Kicking the Inactivity Habit with All the Right Moves

Keep the following in mind as you turn your health and fitness goals into reality by building your exercise plan around activities you prefer.

- ♣ Make sure you see a health professional before you start or modify any plan.
- ♣ Include something to build the following: endurance, strength, and flexibility.
- ♣ Be consistent, and *listen* to your body to avoid injury or health risks. If you're new to exercise, start slow. If you're already doing it, set some new goals and mix up your routine to gain greater balance in the FITT principle we discussed previously.
- ♣ Walk the dog twenty to thirty minutes a day. If you don't have a dog…walk it anyway

Now What? Putting It All Together

First get the go-ahead from your doctor—which may require a stress test and some other body chemistry profiles.

Then, ask around for the names of a fitness trainer. Make an appointment to do a full fitness evaluation (body composition profile, strength/range of motion, and flexibility/cardio health, etc.). Compare your numbers to where your health professional thinks you should be for your age and body type, and have them develop a personal plan to reach and sustain your goals.

Set some realistic goals, and get moving…exercising caution and consistency with the FITT principle.

Have fun, and keep it up.

Now that your transformation of mind and body is nearly complete, the time has come to ensure that you can now afford to live that fuller, healthier lifestyle.

Step #9:
Show Me the Money

On a scale of one to ten, how financially secure or stable do you feel? What would make it a ten? What's your plan to close this gap and preserve or grow what you have?

Like everything else we've discussed and explored so far, financial fitness and security also starts in the mind. Although there is no right financial goal to have, you do have to decide what you want before you can get it. You must understand that your present state of financial strength is nothing more than a manifestation of your previous thinking. Your outer wealth mirrors your inner beliefs.

> "Too many people spend money they haven't earned, to buy things they don't want, to impress people they don't like."
>
> —Will Rogers

Key Smarts and Tools for Financial Survival

There are many facets to consider when creating a financial strategy. In fact, it could be the subject of a whole other book. As you explore and act on the principles in this section, keep in mind that financial freedom is a process, not an event. Five factors should be part of any plan:

- ♣ Decide: How you want to live in the future—your desired lifestyle.
- ♣ Identify: How much you need to live that lifestyle, the gap between what you have and what you will need.
- ♣ Prepare: What's required to get there. Identify ways you can make and save more.
- ♣ Act: On a plan that sets goals and identifies the steps to reach them.
- ♣ Modify: As needed, with the guidance of an expert on such subjects as:
  - Should I start, add to, or modify my retirement account(s)?
  - Do I pay down your mortgage or invest in a new venture or property?
  - Which financial moves may or may not be a good option for you?

When creating your financial goals, remember that there is a life you live now and a life you want to be able to live (afford) in the future. Everything you have to this point is the result of the thoughts and actions you have taken in the past. So getting more and keeping more of what you've already got requires that you become more conscious about your real financial needs, habits, and options. Financial planners call this your financial literacy—and it is the foundation of your "fiscal fitness."

What it means is you know precisely where you are now, exactly where you want to go, and the best path for *you* to get there.

> **"The number one problem in today's generation and economy is the lack of financial literacy."**
> —Alan Greenspan, former Chairman of the Federal Reserve Board

How Strong and Healthy Are Your Finances?

Do you find yourself asking, "If only I had more financial freedom and more income? If only there was a way to enhance my quality of life and improve my financial future?"

Although each generation can ask this question, boomers are more worried about their financial future than at any other time in the past thirty years. Thousands of baby boomers are turning fifty every day. For many of them the question is not when they can retire—it's if they can retire.

Because we're living longer, we need more money to pay for those extra years. There are three financial factors that make or erode your financial worth—and each must be managed from here on out:

- ♠ Income—How much you make with your time, energy, and skill.
- ♠ Outgo—Where it goes, how much, and how often.
- ♠ Equity—What your money does for you…in investments, passive income, etc.

> "Compound interest is the eighth natural wonder of the world and the most powerful thing I have ever encountered."
>
> —Albert Einstein

What Would You Have Left If You Lost Everything?

After years of discipline and hard work, I lost everything I had built over my life for my security. No, I was not "down to only credit cards"...I am talking about losing my dignity, health, self-respect, and being less than a week from living out of my car! After my "financial meltdown," I was looking to rent a room—sadly, all my stuff would have fit in a seven by seven room. *Ouch!* What a financial *mess*, and what a different world from what I had known.

Remember playing Monopoly? Well, this phase in my life wasn't a practice session. It was the real thing; it was *Lifeopoly!*

I asked myself some really tough questions and started looking down a new road. Good news: What took twenty-three years to build the first time was recovered in less than a year. How? *I created my own "luck" with the courage to change my financial literacy with the same tools that you can use.* Luck is the residue of planning!

Outer wealth and security starts with inner wealth and security.

Tools You Can Use

- *New Mindset*: if it's to be it's up to me. Create a strategy to maximize your income, compound your earning potential, and minimize your outgo.
- *New Plan* from a "mentor": learn from the time and experience of those who have what you want.
- *New Focused Action*: apply discipline and consistency to make your plan work. Look into support from resources such as *Start Late, Finish Rich* by David Bach, originator of "The Latté Factor" investment strategy. You decide where your money comes from and goes...*Rich Dad, Poor Dad* by Robert Kiyosaki. The discipline of delayed gratification...*The Millionaire Next Door* by Thomas J. Stanley.

> **"If you are not financially independent by the time you are forty or fifty, it doesn't mean that you are living in the wrong country or at the wrong time. It simply means that you have the wrong plan."**
> —Jim Rohn

One reason most people don't draw or keep financial success into their life is because of their thinking. Always be mindful of and act on the principle "an ounce of prevention is worth a pound of cure."

Financial Wake-up Call— Identity Theft

Okay, you don't think *you* would be as stupid as I was. You have everything under control...or do you? Here's how to keep more of what you have:

- Regularly pull a copy of your credit report.
- Securely store or dispose of your personal papers and financial papers.
- Limit the number of people who have access to your accounts.
- Store your account passwords in a safe place.
- Keep important papers together in a secure location.

No News Is Not Always Good News!

Make sure you review your credit report a couple of times a year for errors and discrepancies that could cost you dearly. For additional information, contact these valuable credit resources:

- Free Annual Credit Reports: www.freeannualcreditreports.com
- Equifax: www.equifax.com
- Experian (formerly TRW): www.experian.com
- TransUnion: www.transunion.com

Additional numbers of interest include:

- 800-5-OPTOUT to cut unsolicited sales calls
- Call for Action—Visa to question charges on a credit card: 877-567-8688
- Privacy Rights Clearing House at www.privacyrights.org

Un-thinkable Frauds Are Real

Internet auction/counterfeit check/overpayment frauds generally occur online, in person, or by mail during the sale of a higher value item, such as a car. What to do to protect yourself:

- Verify payment is legitimate by contacting the buyer's bank before shipping the item.
- Remember that a bank's release of the money does not guarantee the funds are legitimate.
- Avoid giving your bank account or credit card number to unknown parties.

Advanced fee and "lottery" frauds/wiring funds out of the country generally occur by phone or online. If you are contacted as a lottery winner, promised a large payment, and asked to send money for taxes on your winnings or suffer the loss of money you sent, follow these preventive tips!

- Never reply to an email requesting funds or give out personal information.
- Verify that the business or offer is legitimate.
- Be suspicious of any request to withdraw cash and wire funds.

Phone/confidence frauds generally occur by an unsolicited call for a fictitious charity, business or investment. If this happens or you are unsure, do not provide any account or personal information until you have verified the legitimacy of the organization. Ask them to mail you the information instead.

Funding Your Future

Aside from finding a *"trust fund"* baby boomer willing to share their wealth with you, *your* savings and investing habits determine how well you retire.

Financial Security

There are plenty of resources for setting a booming plan for financial freedom. In the book *The Latté Factor*, author David Bach shows the cumulative value of putting aside five dollars a day for ten plus years to "Start" the habit of savings. Although it is not much, it shows the value in setting new spending priorities to accumulate more financial freedom.

> **"Just when I figured out how to make ends meet, they moved the ends."**
> —financial planner's client

Experts recommend aiming toward:

- ⏣ Living on 70%—Learn to pay yourself first, before you pay your monthly bills.
- ⏣ Saving 10%—Set up an automatic deposit to set aside part of what you make.
- ⏣ Giving 10%—Giving back has many rewards—emotional, spiritual, and financial.
- ⏣ Investing 10%—Make more from what you have.

Keep in mind that saving is unnatural for some and that giving is in our DNA. Do some side research to discover which kind of saving, giving, and investing gives you the most value.

Seek out a financial planner that can helps you put together a profitable wealth-preserving/building plan.

Want More Information?

Some helpful resources are:
www.suzeorman.com.
www.cfp.org
www.finishrich.com

Covering Your Asset—
Legal Maneuvers and Insurance

Legal maneuvers. It's easy to say that you don't like law-yers—until you need one. Putting all opinions and kidding aside, there are several ways for you to benefit from their help. Legal awareness and empowerment is a powerful strategy for preserving wealth. It can protect you from life's uncertainties. Marriage, divorce, death, medical issues ill-ness, business issues, your rights —at home, work, or play…we could go on and on, but they each affect your stress load and bank account.

A little bit of pre-planning with a legal specialist in your area of need can reduce or eliminate grief, loss, worry, and tension through better "fiscal fitness." One word of caution…be sure to match you legal beagle to your spe-cific area of need. After all, you wouldn't go to a foot doctor for heart health, would you?

> **"The smart man knows what he doesn't know."**
> **—Proverb**

What's the best bankruptcy action? Get an expert, regardless of what stage you are at:

- ♣ Contemplating…is this the right way to file?
- ♣ In the middle of it…don't screw up.
- ♣ After recovery, feel good about the right road to go down.

After my bankruptcy, I found both information and resources at www.afterbankruptcy.org.

Insurance—Protect What's Yours

Oversights, mistakes, and accidents can create unnecessary loss. A key part of protecting what you have worked hard to create is having the proper type and amount of insurance in place. Unfortunately, many boomers feel the same way about insurance as they do lawyers…until their car gets wrecked, the house floods, or they need to cover other losses or surprises from life.

What type is best? Look at what you want to keep, and find a referral to a professional who can create a policy to protect you from the risk of loss.

Putting It All Together…Exercises for Building a Wealthier You!

Revisit and redefine how you feel about money:

When I was growing up, I was taught that money was

_____.

Today I feel money is _____, and I am okay with this new perception.

Release yourself from the memories that are no longer true for you, and rebuild your beliefs around your current values.

Knowledge is power so whatever your lifestyle calls for, learn about the following areas of financial health and safeguarding:

- Managing debt
- Home ownership
- Insurance
- Paying for college
- Retirement planning

Seek out an expert or book and set up a new financial plan by completing the following steps:

Focus—What is your goal?

Plan—What is your time frame and possible barriers or obstacles?

Decide—How to overcome obstacles and barriers.

Act—With courage and coaching. Financial independence is great....but it's rarely achieved alone.

Consistency—Without momentum, you can't get ahead.

> **The price of success is much lower than the price of regret.**

Step #10:
Doctor, Doctor, Give Me the News!

Although more and more boomers avoid death in our early years, we must still learn how to improve our resistance factors while eliminating risk factors. Becoming well and remaining so means more than seeing a doctor when you're sick. It means becoming aware of the role you play in preventing illness and promoting wellness in your own life not only to preserve your longevity but also to pay for it.

> **"The first wealth is health."**
> —Ralph Waldo Emerson

Many boomers erroneously believe that because they are not sick, they are well. My father's "instant death" from a heart attack (with no history of illness or disease) supports the idea that thinking you are well because you are not sick is misleading and can even be deadly.

According to data compiled by the American Psychiatric and Medical Associations, only five percent of our population as a whole is thriving, while over seventy-five percent of us are not sick but not fully well either.

Using prescription and non-prescription medications to control symptoms may cover them up, but the underlying problem may still exist—and lead to disaster down the road.

Knowledge Is Power—You May Need More Than a Blood Pressure Check

A new branch of medicine, functional medicine, has emerged to help us to focus on prevention as well as intervention in our quest to champion our own health and longevity. Utilizing the array of tests and screenings through this anti-aging team of professionals can prolong life while enhancing quality of life.

If you look at your own health and wellness scale—where are you? Where do you want to be? How to reduce the gap?

Wellness	Health	Disease and Death
The more time and $ here	Less $ spent here	Avoid and slower to get here

What's Your Health Age vs. Your *Body* Age...Take This Test

A longer, better life isn't always based on your genes. It's in your habits. Longevity expert Dr. Michael Roizen says that everyone has two ages: your chronological age and your *real* age. Your real age is determined by your lifestyle rather than your birthday. Visit www.realage.com and take the real age test and find out where you have the most room for improvement. Doing so will help you keep your risk factors from ending up as disease—a lesson learned too late by my father whose death could have been prevented by a trip to a functional medicine physician.

> "You have a healthy body for
> someone twice your age."
> —Anonymous

Maybe It Will Go Away...The Five Most Dangerous Words in Our Boomer Language

As your power years unfold, there are many tools in your wellness support team's arsenal to see if you're making the grade or losing ground. From your teeth and your toes to your spine and your chest, the most basic tests to reveal the impact of your life with a window to your internal world include:

- Tests (through blood, urine, hair, saliva, MRI, ultrasound , radiology, "scopes", etc.) to check your general health or the health of certain parts of your body
- Measurements of weight, body composition profile, cholesterol levels, and blood pressure
- Posture exam and spine alignment assessment
- Dental exams for oral cancer and other health risks associated with your teeth
- Stress assessments and stress management techniques and programs (see below)
- Special tests for hormone levels (see below)
- Nutritional deficiency test and other advancements in science to give you answers

What's the Best Health Insurance?

The best insurance is always prevention instead of intervention. In order to prevent unnecessary medical surprises and their associated costs, see your physician to identify your body's current condition, your risk factors, and a plan to fill the gaps. Talk over which tests you need and how often with your healthcare provider.

Top Ten Signs You Have Joined a Cheap HMO—From Dr. Mark Houston

- Annual breast exam conducted at Hooters.
- Directions to your doctor's office include "take a left when you enter the trailer park."
- Tongue depressors taste faintly of Fudgesicles™.
- Only proctologist in the plan is "Gus" from Roto-Rooter™.
- Only item listed under Preventative Care is "an apple a day."
- Your "primary care physician" is wearing the pants you gave to Goodwill™ last month.
- "Patient responsible for 200% of out-of-network charges" is not a typo.
- The only expense covered 100% is embalming.
- With your last HMO, your Prozac™ didn't come in different colors, with little "m's" on them.
- And the number one sign you've joined a cheap HMO…

You asked for Viagra. You get a Popsicle stick and duct tape!

Stress and the Cortisol Cops...Tests You Can Take to See If Stress Is Harming Your Body

Tired, worn-out, just can't recover from life's demands no matter what you do? Many boomers are feeling so overtired we don't even have the energy to have fun. But why? One possible answer could be adrenal burnout!

One of the most common and overlooked problems facing our generation is adrenal fatigue from a decrease in a hormone called cortisol. Essentially, cortisol protects the body from excess stress. When it is out of balance or lacking, it can lead to adrenal fatigue—kind of like the alternator not working in your car.

According to James L. Wilson, author of *Adrenal Fatigue, the 21st Century Stress Syndrome*, adrenal fatigue (technically called "hypoadrenia" and "hypoadrenalism") has been one of our most prevalent yet rarely diagnosed conditions for the last fifty years. Despite being described in medical texts over one hundred years ago, many physicians are just now becoming aware of why this condition exists and how to treat it.

But There Is Help

In his book Dr. Wilson explains the causes, tests, and treatments for Adrenal Fatigue and your recovery from it. Another resource, *From Fatigue to Fantastic*, by Dr. Jacob Teitelbaum, M.D., shows therapies to overcome this vitality zapping illness as well.

> "I'm not here for advice, Doc, I'm here for more candles..."
> —stress management patient

Natural HRT— The Truth for Women and Men

According to anti-aging experts, our hormones don't decline because we age, we age because our hormones decline. However, there is no one-size-fits-all program for which ones do you take, how often, and for how long. So be sure to see a physician that is board certified in anti-aging medicine to keep yourself hormonally sound.

Attention Women!

Throughout your forties, fifties, sixties, and beyond, your body changes. As your body changes, so do your needs. Fluctuating hormone levels contribute to a host of health and quality-of-life issues and conditions. But don't go it alone or suffer in silence. Get the knowledge and help you need to reclaim your life!

In her book, *HRT: The Answers*, Dr. Pamela Wartian Smith, M.D., MPH, director of the Center for Healthy Living and Longevity, shares that a woman's health is profoundly affected by her body's ability to maintain hormone balance. If her hormonal balance is disrupted, numerous health problems and conditions can follow.

Current research estimates that over 3,500 women in the United States enter menopause each day and that the symptoms can go past the proverbial "hot-flashes." As one of several groundbreaking resources on the subject, Dr. Smith's book helps you gain new awareness on what to do, when, why, and how in order to be more hormonally balanced.

> "I'm still hot...it just comes in flashes."
> —Unknown

Some of the symptoms that you may be going through menopause or that your hormones are out of balance include:

- Aching joints
- Anxiety
- Bloat/Gas
- Depression
- Forgetfulness
- Frequent urination mood swings
- Hair growth on the face
- Hot flashes
- Insomnia
- Indigestion
- Lower back pain
- Night sweats
- Osteoporosis
- Panic attacks
- Sore breasts
- Varicose veins
- Weight gain
- Weird dreams

While certainly not an exhaustive list, it shows how all the hormones in your body are designed to work together. When they are out of balance, a host of annoying physical challenges can occur.

Other resources to solve the HRT challenge for women include: www.biohrt.com (Natural HRT for Women).

Another organization and resource to help you keep on top of your game is the National Association of Baby Boomer Women (www.nabbw.com). NABBW is dedicated to empowering women to explore their passions and live life to the fullest. Through their organization, website and a "must-have" electronic newsletter, *Boomer Women Speak* (www.boomerwomenspeak.com), they connect, encourage, and support the interests and needs of baby boomer women everywhere. With over sixty forums (on everything from empty nest and step-children to menopause and caring for your parents) you're sure to find what you need to be informed, empowered, and renewed on your journey as a boomer woman.

> "Never go to a doctor whose house plants have died."
> —Erma Bombeck

Men's Health—
Time Out for Testosterone

According to longevity experts, hormone replacement therapy for men is just as important as hormone replacement for women. Labeled the "sex drive" hormone, testosterone levels drop about one percent per year starting around age thirty, This "male menopause" or *andropause* becomes more apparent in men around age fifty. Studies show cardiovascular, cognitive, and other benefits improve when aging men are given hormone supplementation. The following list can show if you may want to talk to your doctor about whether natural hormone replacement therapy is something for you to consider.

Signs You May Need A Testosterone Tune-Up

- Fatigue
- Tiredness
- Loss of drive and competitive edge

- Depression, mood changes
- Falling levels of fitness
- Stiffness in muscles and joints
- Reduced libido (desire for sex)
- Loss of muscle, more fat

This is only a partial list. For a complete list you will want to see a physician board certified in anti-aging and functional medicine.

Dental Diligence—How It Could Save Your Life!

The condition of the mouth mirrors the condition of the body. Today's dental professional is armed with the tools and knowledge to provide you with more than just filling cavities and teeth whitening. Your dentist can identify symptoms associated with some serious medical problems—making them a key ally in detecting, treating, and preventing your health risks early enough to change the outcome.

According to the Michigan Dental Association, your dentist can help in screening for mouth cancer and discovering oral symptoms of diabetes and heart attack or stroke. If any suspect symptoms are found, your dentist can then coordinate a treatment plan with the rest of your wellness team. They can also keep you healthy and happy by identifying the cause and treatment for headaches from TMJ (temporomandibular joint) disorders.

By the way, while we are discussing teeth, a dentist recently told one of my colleagues that the boomer generation's dental habits make us the first generation not obligated to get dentures.

Oh, My Aching Back, Leg, Head...Pain Management

The stress of pain has a huge impact on the aging process. In the same way that leaving your car lights on drains its battery, chronic (long-term) pain from the following conditions zaps your energy and steals your quality of life:

- ♠ Chronic lower back pain.
- ♠ Chronic head and neck pain, including TMJ syndrome.
- ♠ Post-traumatic injuries to extremities.
- ♠ Chronic arthritic and other musculoskeletal pain.
- ♠ Fibromyalgia and other diffuse pain syndromes.
- ♠ Chronic degenerative joint and disk disease.
- ♠ Chronic and acute cancer pain.

But don't despair. Today's pain practitioner has more than pills to treat this multiplicity of ailments and pain conditions and to return you to a more enjoyable life. Your new arsenal of options includes:

- ♠ Spinal cord stimulators implants
- ♠ Multi-agent infusion implant pumps
- ♠ Non-invasive disc decompression therapies
- ♠ Radio frequency treatments
- ♠ Ultrasound guided peripheral nerve stimulators

Other resources for pain management education include: *Easing the Pain of Arthritis Naturally* by Earl Mindell, R.Ph., PhD.

Now What? Putting It All Together

You are officially armed and ready to dream big and live the life you were intended to live. I have done my best to provide you with the insights and tools you need to bring a new level of joy, relevance, and value to your boomer years.

You can't do everything at once, but you can do something each day to close the gap between where you are and where you want to be. Those who previewed this book before its publication to the general pubic said they simply went back to section one, defined some goals, took a couple of new steps, and created a plan that built some incredible momentum toward what they wanted from both life and business.

You can do the same. Take whatever you have learned from this book and apply it. How can you eat better? How can you think better or be more active? How can you deepen your relationships and build your financial freedom? What needs to go and what needs to be added back into your life? What's the vision for your future, why is it important to you, and how will you get there?

You Can't Do Everything at Once, but You Can Begin

I encourage you to revisit this book often. Re-read a section and underline things that are important to you. Doing so will not only reinforce what you already know; you may also discover something new, which didn't register during your first review.

I also encourage you to share this book and what you have learned with your colleagues, friends, and family— even your healthcare provider. One of my clients told me that he wanted this to be *"required reading for my staff and a must-have book for my patients."* I believe that the gift of empowerment is the greatest gift we can share. We all deserve to move past our limits with new thoughts, ideas, and resources for getting more and losing less from life. The key is to take action and get started, from wherever you are.

> **"When the student is ready, the teacher will appear."**
> —Proverb

The Journey Continues...

Your life is a gift. The secret to how well it's lived does not come from your genes...it comes from your head, hands, and heart! Most of the things that cause us the most grief are usually our own doing.

Don't waste what you've been given. Get started on the next stage of your life journey...*today!*

Think about how you want your future to play out.

Do something new each day to make that happen.

Be the change you want to see in others—live, love, and laugh—and watch your life go from "survive" to *thrive!*

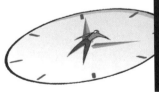

Time Is Your Enemy, or Time Is Your Friend: Which Will It Be for You?

> **"When I told my doctor I couldn't afford an operation, he offered to touch-up my X-rays."**
> —Henny Youngman

Appendix 1:
The Glycemic Index of Foods

What's the Glycemic Index? It's a ranking of carbohydrates based on their immediate impact on your blood sugar. Those that break down quickly during digestion have the highest glycemic index because the blood glucose response is fast and high. Carbohydrates that break down slowly, gradually releasing sugar into your bloodstream, are given a low glycemic index. This chart, although limited, is adapted from the *American Journal of Clinical Nutrition* to guide you in your choices as to which foods you want to include in your diet. Keep in mind that this is not a list of "bad foods," only a guide to foods you may need to limit or avoid from time to time to maintain a healthier insulin response—which ultimately lowers your health risks.

Low GI foods help to:
- ◑ Reduce spikes in blood sugar after meals
- ◑ Improve the body's sensitivity to insulin
- ◑ Re-fuel your body's energy stores after exercise
- ◑ Keep you full longer, so you fill up not *out*!
- ◑ Prolong physical endurance

High Glycemic-Index Foods

- Cookies
- Pasta
- Buns—hotdog and hamburger
- English muffin
- Macaroni and cheese, boxed
- Crackers—corn and wheat thins
- Rolls
- Chips—all kinds
- French fries
- Popcorn
- Breakfast cereals
- Waffles
- Donuts
- Bagels
- Dried fruit
- Honey
- Melba toast
- Rice cakes
- Rice pasta
- Semolina
- Rye flour
- Candy
- Soft drinks
- Pineapple
- Carrots
- Broad beans
- Raisins
- Potatoes
- Watermelon

Moderate Glycemic-Index Foods

- Buckwheat
- Spaghetti, durum
- Pizza with cheese
- Instant noodles
- Orange juice
- Kiwi fruit
- Canned fruits
- Mango
- Chocolate
- Banana
- Blueberry
- "Special K" cereal
- Green peas
- Linguine
- Yams
- Corn
- Roman beans
- Macaroni
- Potato chips

Low Glycemic-Index Foods

- All-bran cereal
- Apples
- Apricots
- Peaches
- Grapefruit
- Plums
- Cherries
- Grapes
- Oranges
- Rice bran
- Soybeans
- Chick peas
- Corn hominy
- Green beans
- Black beans
- Butter beans
- Lentils
- Spaghetti, whole wheat
- Lima beans

Other resources include:

The New Glucose Revolution:
Shopper's Guide to GI Values 2006

The New Glucose Revolution:
People with Diabetes

Appendix 2:
Anti-Aging Recipes

Whether you are a simple eater and prefer dishes that take a few minutes to prepare or a gourmet with a flair for unique and exotic dishes that require more time to get ready, you will find something to please your taste buds within the next few pages.

The recipes that follow have been designed to give you energy and health—the energy and health you need to feel your best at all times.

You will notice as you read through this section that the primary seasonings are herbs and spices—and very little if any salt or sweeteners. We have found that there are many new tastes that can be created without salt or sugar. Don't be afraid to experiment, as these are only a few ideas to get you started. We've included an herb and spice chart in the back to serve as your guide to creating a change in your food preparation methods.

Basic Food Preparation

The preparation of food is a key factor to consider when looking for ways to tip Father Time and the scale in your favor. Aside from frequency and amount, your preparation habits will influence the nutrition you gain per serving.

The best rule of thumb is, "less is more." Too much peeling, cooking, washing, reheating, etc. causes your food to lose valuable nutrients that control your appetite and anti-aging factors. Heat, air, light, and storage each influence the nutrients available to your body from the food you eat.

Keep these tips in mind when preparing and cooking your meals:

Preparation

- If possible, cut foods just prior to use.
- Avoid soaking food in hot water or in containers.
- Use lemon as an anti-oxidation additive to help prevent the discoloration of fruits and vegetables.
- Cut foods in uniform shape and size for even cooking.
- Wash all fruits and vegetables thoroughly with light detergent, with skin on, to remove waxes, dirt, and chemicals.
- If wax or chemicals remain, peel and discard the outer skin.

Cooking

- The best techniques to reduce calories and retain nutrients are: rapid boil, steam, stir-fry, sauté with vegetable spray, braise (very hot, then moderately hot temperature to seal in juices), stew, slow cook, broil.
- When boiling foods, be sure water is brought to a rapid boil before adding vegetables, etc.
- When steaming, put the slowest cooking vegetables on the bottom and the fastest cooking on top.
- When using the stir-fry method, start with the slowest cooking vegetables and meats first, adding vegetables and meats in order of their cooking time.

♠ Keep foods moist by adding stock or vegetable juices during cooking period.

♠ Use fresh vegetables whenever possible. Then opt for fresh froze to ensure optimal taste and nutritional value.

♠ For tender, crisp vegetables—and to retain the natural flavors and nutrients—cook your vegetables in the least amount of water possible in a covered saucepan (or stir-fry in a skillet or wok).

♠ Use vegetable oils in dressings and vegetable sprays when heat is involved.

♠ Season with various vinegars and herbs or spices. Fresh vegetables and meat, poultry, and fish have their own unique and wonderful flavors; season subtly and sparingly. This will enhance instead of cover up their full range of flavor.

♠ Use sauces and dressings sparingly. Choose a sauce or dressing that will compliment the flavor, not cover it up.

Ideas for Quick and Healthy Meals
Breakfast

Better Oats *(serves 1)*

Cook your oats in ½ apple juice and ½ water and add 1/8 t ground cinnamon. That will give it a natural sweetness and new flavor as well as reduce the need for sugar. Using "cultured" milk or yogurt on top makes this a complete protein for breakfast.

Energy Omelet *(serves 1)*

6 ounces cooked fish or poultry
1 cup fresh vegetables
 (peppers, mushrooms, zucchini, broccoli, etc.)
2 large eggs (one yolk only)
2–3 T tomato sauce or Italian salad dressing
¼ t ground ginger
¼ t of your choice: tarragon, cilantro, garlic

Coat medium sauté pan with non-stick spray, and pre-heat pan on high setting on stove. Separately, in medium bowl, whip eggs with spices. Add fish or fowl. Sauté and serve.

Breakfast Brightener Salad *(serves 2)*

1 apple (grated with skin on)
juice of ½ lemon
1 whole kiwi fruit, peeled and sliced
1 whole peach, pitted and diced
½ cup ricotta cheese
1 t honey or molasses
dash of ground cinnamon
1 teaspoon fresh ground ginger (optional)

In small bowl, mix ricotta cheese with honey and cinnamon. Separately mix remaining ingredients and let sit for 3–5 minutes for flavors to blend. Place ½ of ricotta on two plates. Top each plate with ½ of fruit. Serve.

Lunch

Tarragon Tuna Salad *(serves 1)*

¾ cup white Albacore tuna, drained
¼ teaspoon tarragon
2 green onions, chopped
juice of ¼ lemon
3 T balsamic vinegar salad dressing
½ fresh chopped tomatoes
2-3 cups mixed salad greens

Combine tuna with balsamic vinegar, lemon, and tarragon. Mix well, making sure all tuna chunks are broken down (but not mushy) and blended well with liquids. Add onions and tomatoes. Mix lightly. Serve over bed of salad greens. If desired, drizzle extra balsamic dressing over top of salad.

Italian Chicken Salad

Add a mixture of ½ cup chicken and ½ t Italian Seasonings, to salad greens

Tempting Turkey Toss

Add fresh cooked turkey (instead of lunch meat) with shredded zucchini to your salads

Dinner

Spicy Quick Pan-Baked Whitefish *(serves 2)*

2 ounces water
2 eight-ounce white fish filets
2 T Italian Dressing
2 T chopped tomatoes
2–3 green onions, chopped fine

juice of ½ lemon
½ teaspoon dill or tarragon
Non-stick vegetable spray
4–5 drops liquid pepper sauce
(Tabasco, etc.)

Rinse fish and pat dry. Combine all wet and dry ingredients and set aside. Coat medium sauté pan with non-stick spray. Pre-heat pan on high setting, but don't let pan coating "smoke." Add filets and cook 1 minute. Add remaining ingredients and cover. Reduce heat to medium and cook until fish is flaky (about 5 minutes). Serve.

Gingered Southwest Pan-Baked Salmon *(serves 2)*

2 ounces water
2 eight-ounce salmon filets
1 T balsamic vinegar
1 T molasses
1/8 t ground pepper

juice of ½ lime
½ teaspoon fresh grated ginger
Non-stick vegetable spray
1 clove garlic, smashed
2 T orange juice

Rinse fish and pat dry. Combine all wet (except orange juice) and dry ingredients and set aside. Coat medium sauté pan with non-stick spray. Pre-heat pan on high setting, but don't let pan coating "smoke." Add filets and brown one side. Turn them over and add remaining ingredients and cover. Reduce heat to medium and cook until fish is flaky (about 5 minutes). Remove fish from pan. Add orange juice. Continue to cook liquids in the pan to a thick consistency and serve as a sauce over fish.

Turkey/Zucchini Patties *(serves 2)*

1 pound fresh ground turkey	1 t "Mrs. Dash"
½ cup shredded zucchini	3 T balsamic vinegar
2 T Italian dressing	Non-stick vegetable spray
1/8 t ground nutmeg	2 green onions chopped fine

Coat medium sauté pan with spray. Preheat pan over high, but don't let it "smoke." Separately, mix all ingredients well in a medium bowl. Form mixture into two to four patties. Brown each side. Reduce heat and cover. Cook 3–5 more minutes until done. Serve.

Beverage/Snack Ideas

Instant Vitamin C Drink

Combine 1 cup rosehips tea and your favorite juice with ¼ fresh squeezed lemon. Chill and serve.

Sensational Smoothie

In blender, combine: 1 cup of mixed berries, ¼ t cinnamon, 1 t honey, and 6 ounces plain yogurt. Blend for 30 seconds at high speed. Serve.

Fruit Fizzler

Combine 1/3 sparkling water with 2/3 fresh juice of your choice. Chill with frozen fruit pieces.

Parfait

Fill glasses with alternate layers of vanilla yogurt, granola, and fresh fruit. Top with applesauce and fresh strawberries or blueberries.

Better Gelatin Dessert

Make your gelatin dessert with unflavored gelatin and juice, adding fresh fruit for additional flavor and fiber.

Index

Give the Gift of

Baby Boomers Almanac
to Your Friends and Colleagues

CHECK YOUR LEADING BOOKSTORE OR ORDER HERE

❏ **YES**, I want _____ copies of *Baby Boomers Almanac* at $14.95 each, plus $4.95 shipping per book (Michigan residents please add 90¢ sales tax per book). Canadian orders must be accompanied by a postal money order in U.S. funds. Allow 15 days for delivery.

My check or money order for $_____ is enclosed.

Please charge my ❏ Visa ❏ MasterCard ❏ Discover ❏ American Express

Name_____

Organization_____

Address _____

City/State/Zip _____

Phone_____ Email _____

Card # _____

Exp. Date_____ Signature _____

Please make your check payable and return to:

Better Living Publishing
Suite A, 45838 Rapids Drive • Macomb Twp, MI 48044

Fax your credit card order to 586-228-1909

or order online at
www.betterlivingpublishing.com

Want to be part of the
Baby Boomer Movement?

Visit us at www.abetterboomerlife.com for more information.

When you visit us, be sure to tell us how the *Baby Boomers Almanac* has helped you to create greater health, wealth or wisdom.